Falling
Leaf
Essences

Falling Leaf Essences

VIBRATIONAL REMEDIES
USING AUTUMN LEAVES

GRANT R. LAMBERT, PH.D.

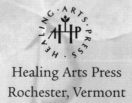

Healing Arts Press
Rochester, Vermont

Healing Arts Press
One Park Street
Rochester, Vermont 05767
www.InnerTraditions.com

Healing Arts Press is a division of Inner Traditions International

LIBRARY OF CONGRESS CATALOGING-IN-PUBLICATION DATA
Lambert, Grant R.
Falling leaf essences : vibrational remedies using autumn leaves /
Grant R. Lambert.
p. cm.
Includes bibliographical references and index.
ISBN 0-89281-928-6
1. Leaves—Therapeutic use. 2. Vibration (Therapeutics) 3. Essences
and essential oils—Therapeutic use. I. Title.
RZ999 .L18 2002
2002002994

Printed and bound in the United States at Lake Book

10   9   8   7   6   5   4   3   2   1

Text design and layout by Virginia L. Scott Bowman
This book was typeset in Legacy Serif and Legacy Sans with
Highlander as the display typeface

Contents

Fallen Leaves

You apple tree you stand so still,
Naked now against the chill,
Yet again, quite unasked,
You've shed your leaves, uncloaked, unmasked.
These fallen leaves lay at your feet,
Slowly fading, their work complete,
And you in your wisdom are not one who clings
To what has been, outgrown things.
Barren and dormant, quietly you sleep,
Peaceful, accepting, you do not weep,
With the coming of spring you emerge cleansed and
    whole,
And bear once again the fruit of your soul.
As day turns to darkness and darkness to light,
So you flow with all changes, you put up no fight,
Your grace at all times, your ease to just be,
Has so much to teach us, you apple tree.

Marilyn Butt

Preface: Advanced Alchemy

THIS BOOK REPRESENTS THE DISTILLATION of about a decade of thought and research centered on healing and essences. I began working on the conceptual basis for the development of new essence categories in 1988; the actual work in making the falling leaf essences began in 1994. These projects have fascinated, intrigued, and absorbed me such that I never seriously questioned the appropriateness of getting involved in them. From the outset, I have had a strong sense that both the conceptual and practical aspects of falling leaf essences are an essential part of my life journey. Many thousands of hours have gone into these projects over that decade of time.

There are two different aspects of essences that continue to intrigue me. The first is their potential as relatively safe, inexpensive, and powerful agents in healing. This aspect will be developed fully in this book. The second is their existence in the first place. According to the worldview of materialistic science, essences ought not to exist. I am faced with the curious contradiction that I have spent the past fifteen years exploring in detail a phenomenon that does not exist according to the establishment! Either I have spent a decade and a half wandering in a fantastically detailed and consistent but completely imaginary world, or in fact essences do exist. If essences do exist, then the implications for science and for our concept of the world, how it came to be, and our place within it all go through a considerable revolution. The manner in which our emerging understanding of essences changes our view of the universe and of ourselves might indeed be the topic for a future book.

As I reflect upon this work about the falling leaf essences, four aspects stand out in my mind. The first is the immense enjoyment I have derived from both the conceptual and the practical aspects of falling leaf essences. They have given me many unforgettable moments of magic. I will never forget the first color diagrams of falling leaf essence action that I drew, on a card table set up in the garden in spring, the sun filtering through the trees above. It was a moment in which the quality of the environment and the thrill of creativity expressed in color came together in a kind of ecstasy. Years later, I am still excited and amazed by the thought of it. Wonder and magic also surround the trip to Bright in 1994, which I describe in chapter 3 of this book. Words somehow fall far short of describing the sense of spiritual purpose and unity with nature and spirit that descended upon me in that place. A third emotionally evocative image is of the Oak Lawn at the Royal Botanical Gardens in Melbourne, Australia, in autumn. The Royal Botanical Gardens has a magnificent array of mature oak trees. As I was collecting specimens of fallen oak leaves one autumn, a group of schoolchildren on a field trip were playing on the carpet of fallen leaves. As they played, picking up handfuls of leaves and scattering them in gay abandon, a wonderful union began to take place. It was as if these children, in the "spring" of their life, were joining together in an ecstatic dance with the autumn leaves. Spring and autumn became one; it seemed as if the leaves danced of their own accord with the children. I remember this experience as "the dance of the falling leaves."

The second memorable aspect of the falling leaf project has been the assistance it has given me in restoring my own creativity. Unfortunately, in order to become educated and then highly educated, it became necessary for me to suppress key aspects of my own thinking and my own being. [Although I value my education and what I have gained from it, the downside was the need to conform to the teachers' way of thinking in order to get top marks. The few times that I expressed what I really thought, I was punished severely by the examiners' marks, which ensured even greater suppression and conformity.]

By the time I became a university student in the mid-1970s, I had developed a coping mechanism that enabled me to attain a bachelor's degree in biochemistry and subsequently a Ph.D. in the same field from the Australian National University in Canberra, at twenty-four years of age. I now look upon that coping mechanism as a kind of "intellectual schizophrenia." It consisted of regurgitating back to professors exactly what they wanted to hear or read and keeping my own thinking and interpretation entirely inner, unspoken, and unwritten. To think that the pressure to conform was any less when I was a doctoral student as when I was an undergraduate would be entirely delusional.

The stress of maintaining this intellectual schizophrenia was probably one of the triggers for the chronic fatigue syndrome from which I suffered from 1983 through 1987. This illness, and my recovery from it, brought many changes in my life. One certainty that emerged was that I would not go back to work in a university environment again. For a young, successful scientist who had been the primary author on scientific papers published in journals as prestigious as the *Proceedings of the National Academy of Science,* this was a bittersweet pill to swallow. The sweet aspect was that, being no longer employed by a university, I was actually free to think and express myself as I wanted.

Thus I began my studies in natural therapies and, in particular, homeopathy, which had been instrumental in my recovery from chronic fatigue syndrome. I soon found that healing was a fascinating realm for the development of ideas, concepts, and new treatments. It has certainly taken many years for me to gain the courage and conviction to venture forth openly with my ideas. I keep expecting the familiar heavy rod of punishment, even when nowadays I search for it in vain. I do not find punishment, but I do find a great deal of apathy and apparent refusal to think about the healing process and essences in particular. It is no secret that as an inventor of new ideas and products in the realm of essences, one meets enormous resistance.

The first time that I spoke publicly to a group of people concerning falling leaf essences was a thrilling, engaging, stimulating, and terrifying experience. Having acquitted myself admirably on the day, I then proceeded to undergo several weeks of intense inner change. It felt as though taking that which for decades had been inner, secret, unspoken, and unwritten and proclaiming it openly, like a trumpeter from a public platform, was enough to turn me upside down and inside out.

Third, the work presented in this book has been extremely demanding on many levels. To omit this point would be to impart an imbalanced picture of the situation. The vast majority of research projects in the modern era are funded either by governments or by large corporations. As a research scientist, I have worked under both such funding arrangements. The problem with either situation is that the body controlling the purse strings also controls the research. The controlling body generally requires that regular reports be submitted in order for the worthiness of giving future funding to the project to be assessed. On one level, this might be considered simply good financial management. On another level, it can be quite a diabolical manipulation. What's assessed is not just whether progress is being made, but also whether this progress is to the ideological or economic liking of the funding body.

Legion are the scientific projects that have been terminated because they were tending in the direction of new paradigms or findings contrary to the ideological foundations of the prevailing system, or toward new inventions that were contrary to the interests of the system. Likewise, the life of a research scientist is analogous to that of a politician; both must impress their electorate by pursuing short-term rather than long-term goals.

I did not believe that the research project described in this book could have attracted funding from any government or corporation in existence at the time. It was simply too far removed from prevalent thinking in medicine and healing. Moreover, having experienced funded research programs and the web of control they weave, I was aware from the outset that these projects *had to be* free of such control. This, I believe, is a profound gift to the readers of the book: the knowledge that the ideas and research presented are exactly as I conceived them to be. There is no place where I "follow the party line" or say anything other than what I really mean in order to conform to any external ideological or financial pressure.

It is a rare privilege to be able to have such purity of intent and communication in the dollar-driven era in which we live. On the other hand, the price of ideological freedom can be a loss of economic well-being and freedom. In the extreme case, total ideological freedom exists in an environment of total poverty. As the cost of the falling leaf and other essence research has multiplied in recent years, it has become increasingly difficult to fund this from personal resources. My response to this ongoing financial pressure has been to see more clients and work more hours in my healing practice. I sometimes find myself working all day with clients to generate the funds to work all night on the essence and writing projects. In such a situation, one finds oneself on the horns of a dilemma—but this dilemma is so familiar to me as to provoke nothing more than a yawn. I needed to do these projects without outside funding, and I am glad to have done so, but this path is not sustainable in the long term.

The life of a private inventor represents an inverted reality with respect to most other professions. In most professions, the harder you work, the more you are paid. As an inventor, the harder you work, the more you pay. One really needs a sizable inheritance, a second profession that enables one to earn large sums of money in short periods of time (such as being a bank robber), or a few significant lottery wins to stay afloat.

Inventive work in the realm of healing and essences is also demanding with respect to the psychic energies involved. Some people would understand these difficult psychic energies as the action of invisible spiritual beings that act to oppose the progress of humanity. Others would understand these energetic difficulties as constituting the reaction of the collective unconscious of humanity, with its resistance to change and growth. Whatever theoretical, theological, or philosophical framework is invoked to explain these energies, in practice they do take their toll. There are days when the need to deal with these extraneous invisible energies halts progress in the visible realm. New Age solutions to these psychic energies, such as surrounding oneself with white light or believing only in Love and Light, abound. I wish they worked. However, surrounding oneself with white light in order to fend off these extreme psychic energies is analogous to expecting an umbrella to protect one in the face of an avalanche. The reality is that working with new inventions in healing and alchemy stirs up these psychic energies on an ongoing basis, and the level of psychic phenomena far exceeds what one would ever experience in "normal" day-to-day living. In fact, I have often noted that the importance of an invention can be fairly accurately ascertained from the level of psychic intensity that accompanies it.

In my early days as an inventor, I was sufficiently naive as to believe that society actually wanted cures for its most common medical ills. This gullibility was the source of many disappointments. One must realize that once society recognizes an illness syndrome and names it, over time that syndrome becomes institutionalized. Doctors, specialists, nurses, research departments, support groups—sometimes even entire hospitals and outpatient wings—all spring up, devoted to treating this illness syndrome. It sometimes seems as though these institutions and trained medical people, although called forth by the best of motives, begin to feed off the illness syndrome for their own livelihood. In other words, these institutions exist both to treat and to perpetuate the diagnosis, treatment, and research of the illness syndrome. If an effective cure for the illness were found, it would render these institutions and personnel redundant overnight. [It is a curious paradox that healers and institutions called forth by the best of motives can on another, unconscious level be involved in continuing and even protecting the illness syndrome that they consciously are devoted to curing or at least ameliorating.]

Only by understanding this am I able to comprehend the rejection and outright hostility that can greet new medical invention, particularly that which is developed "outside the system." There was a time when I felt acutely the pain of those suffering from different illnesses. However, having experienced rejection and hostility from institutions, groups, and people claiming to be working toward the betterment of those suffering from these illnesses, I recognized that the perpetuation of these illnesses was a choice that certain people were making. Both people who are actually ill and groups seeking to help them can have an unconscious need for illness, which manifests as a resistance to any truly effective therapy. Alternatively, ill people and assisting groups can reject any cure that does not conform to their preexisting ideological framework around healing. Such "tunnel vision" might eliminate a range of excellent possibilities, essences included. I shed tears for them. It may not have done them any good, but it did me good. I no longer felt their pain, and I was able to see that the pain was a choice that they had made at some unconscious level.

An equally frustrating picture is that presented by some natural therapists in Australia who use homeopathy or Bach flower remedies. These therapists can be so locked into the mind-set of a bygone era that they continue in a therapeutic vein as if the past century or two simply hadn't happened. In my career as a research scientist, it was absolutely imperative to keep up with the latest developments and the relevant literature. All the research scientists I worked with, in Australia, England, and the United States, were well aware of the fact that time and energy had to be allocated to remain contemporary. I simply do not understand the prevalence in Australia of natural therapists who not only do not keep up with developments in their fields but, moreover, see no need to do so.

As the old saying goes, you can lead a horse to water, but you can't make it drink. Every new idea and invention has its window of opportunity in history. If introduced too early or too late, it goes unheeded and unrecognized. In contrast with the depressing picture painted above, I do believe that the time for falling leaf essences is at hand. There is at least an openness and receptivity to new essences among a subsection of the general population.

A consistent trend that I have observed over the past decade is that clients have an increased level of insight as to the factors underlying their own illnesses. It is indeed rare for me to interact with a client who has no idea what underlies his or her condition. [The days of expecting a practitioner to come up with a pill or potion so that the patient can continue the lifestyle that generated the problem in the first place are receding. (And really, that was an absurd proposition from the outset.)] These increased levels of awareness show that the time for a better understanding of healing is at hand. Likewise, the very language that I hear clients use, that they need to "release" something or "let go," calls to mind the very nature of falling leaf essences.

Fourth, a delightful aspect of the work has been the teamwork, interaction, and cooperation that has enabled the work to progress. Prominent writer Robert Lawlor encouraged me many years ago to further develop and present my ideas. In terms of the actual development of falling leaf essences, two people have played an important role. Both Trudi Dempsey and Jennie Richardson have been clients of my healing practice who showed a particular aptitude and passion for essence research. After I conceived the idea of the essences in Bright, Trudi and I worked together, collecting leaves, identifying them, and intuiting their actions. The methodical approach that Trudi brought to the work from her years of experience in computing was much appreciated. Jennie not only has been involved in these activities in recent years, but also has taken responsibility for the storage of the essences and the numerous day-to-day tasks involved in managing an essence work. Jennie is not only a qualified kinesiologist, but has a deep relationship with nature and with essences as well.

In 1997 I formed the company Advanced Alchemy Pty. Ltd. The primary goal of Advanced Alchemy is to research, develop, and communicate new types of essences toward the end of fostering greater peace and harmony in individuals and in the world in which we live. The vision of Advanced Alchemy has to do not only with essences as products but also with developing appropriate philosophy and models around essences, including understanding essences themselves. In a sense, an essence is either empowered or disempowered by the ideological framework surrounding it. The heart of Advanced Alchemy is the nature philosophy that will be expounded in this book. Advanced Alchemy is also founded on definite standards for essence research and testing, which probably stem from my scientific background.

My wife, Barbara, has been a quiet but keen supporter of the essence work from the beginning and has participated in the sacrifices that it has entailed. My thanks are extended to the therapists described in this book, who have offered themselves and their unwitting clients on the altar of sacrifice in order to test these new remedies. Libby Gordon has worked tirelessly both as a practitioner of these new essences and as the primary teacher and educator of Advanced Alchemy Pty. Ltd. Finally, the belief and enthusiasm that Ehud Sperling, Jeanie Levitan, and Jon Graham of Healing Arts Press have expressed for the *Falling Leaf Essences* manuscript have been most encouraging.

1 The World of Essences

A CHARACTERISTIC FEATURE OF THE INTRODUCTION of new remedies in natural medicine in the modern era is excessive promotion. Great waves of popularity for new products sweep the Western world, while the accumulated knowledge and understanding of thousands of valuable natural remedies is seemingly forgotten for the sake of novelty. Perhaps there exists within the human psyche an unsatisfied quest for the universal remedy, the cure-all that is both the fountain of youth and the Holy Grail. As we may infer from the flurries of advertising that promote this ongoing crusade, it appears that the universal panacea should be capable not only of curing all health problems, but also of delivering joy, happiness, and abundant energy on an indefinite basis. It appears that people tend to want to believe in wonder drugs that will fulfill their unmet physical and emotional needs regardless of the actual effects of those substances on their health and well-being. For decades, cigarettes were promoted on a "they'll make you feel good" basis similar to that used today for modern natural health potions.

An observer of this process might well conclude that promotion and understanding are inversely related. That is, the more imbalanced or deficient the understanding of a particular remedy, the greater the promotion required to overcome this deficit.

In reality, the full spectrum of natural remedies, including aloe vera, ginseng, evening primrose oil, shark cartilage, homeopathics, and noni juice, to mention but a few, are all good products, but each has strengths and weaknesses. Using any such substance or group of substances as a cure-all is bound ultimately to generate disillusionment, because it is an illusion from the outset to believe that any substance is best for everything. A more mature approach, which exists, I hope, at least at the practitioner level, is to integrate new substances into a broader therapeutic picture that recognizes areas of strength and areas of weakness inherent in each prescriptive option.

This book explores falling leaf essences, a group of essences that are fundamentally different from those commonly available today. It is an incredibly exciting discovery to find that in the falling leaf essences there is a majestic healing power around the theme of releasing the old and letting go of the past. Those very aspects of your own past, mentally, emotionally, and physically, that you never seemed able to quite overcome or to effectively release, now can be addressed. These new essences are subtle, yet so incredibly powerful. At times, you will feel them at work on your physical body, encouraging detoxification and release. At other times, they will make themselves known to you in your dreams, with a collage of people and events from the recent and distant past. The emotions and memories of days gone by will again fill your consciousness with a powerful awareness that this is indeed a final letting go, a potent cleansing. In all of this, the falling leaf essences will thwart your best efforts to resist them, and you will move toward becoming the person you always dreamed of being. But as impressed as I am with their capacity for healing, I would not naively claim that these essences are a cure-all—this being the type of notion that we have just discredited. I seek instead to help you develop an understanding of their particular strengths and weaknesses. When will falling leaf essences be most appropriate, and when will a homeopathic or flower essence be more relevant or suitable? What are the guiding principles for the selection of different types of essences? Do these principles lead us only to falling leaf essences or to other new types of essence as well? How do we make and store these new essences, and what can they accomplish in practice?

These questions presuppose an understanding of other types of essences. This understanding is essential and forms the context or landscape within which falling leaf essences can be placed. This chapter seeks to develop a basic understanding of the different types of essences, which is a fascinating subject in its own right.

A Brief History of Modern Medicine

The twentieth century may well be remembered for three very significant advances in medicine. The first is the advent of pharmacology, or modern drug-based medicine, and the phenomenal progress and proliferation of pharmaceuticals since the 1950s. The second is the technological explosion, which has revolutionized both diagnostics and surgery. The third is the incredible growth of interest in methods of healing loosely grouped under the term *natural remedies,* such as herbs, vitamins, minerals, homeopathics, and flower essences.

Arguably, the progress in technology, which manifests in laser surgery, detailed blood tests, CAT scans, and so on, is virtually unlimited in its potential for further development. However, the heyday of pharmaceutical medicine may have been in the 1960s, '70s, and '80s. Although new pharmaceuticals continue to enter the market, there are fewer new introductions than in previous decades. Pharmaceutical medicine is invaluable and indispensable, yet we see indications that there are limits to what it can achieve. It is also doubtful that there exists an unlimited supply of novel, effective medications yet to be discovered. Members of the medical profession certainly do appear to have become more polished and refined in their prescription of existing pharmaceuticals over time.

While pharmaceuticals have occupied the center stage of prescriptive medicine for the second half of the twentieth century, increasing attention is being paid to other branches of prescriptive medicine. It appears that natural remedies, including herbal medicine, homeopathy, and flower essences, work reasonably well. Increasingly, scientific studies support their effectiveness, although the purists can always fault aspects of these.

Herbal medicine is not far removed from pharmaceutical medicine in some respects. Indeed, many modern pharmaceuticals were at least initially derived from plants, although now they are synthetically manufactured. In this way there was a logical progression from herbal to pharmaceutical medicine. However, herbalism and pharmaceutical medicine have very different philosophical platforms. In brief, herbalists argue that the whole is greater than the sum of its parts; that is, herbal preparations made from the whole plant or from one of its parts have an innate balance that benefits the human who ingests them. By contrast, pharmaceutical medicine argues that only the pharmacologically active ingredient need be used. It is believed that the rest of the herb is at best unnecessary and at worst may contain toxins or compounds that are harmful to the human system.

Herbal medicine and pharmacology do share a common presupposition of material science, which is that biological activity can be ascribed to the presence of biologically active molecules or atoms in the prescriptive substance. By contrast, other branches of prescriptive medicine, such as homoeopathy and flower essences, depart altogether from the above-defined materialistic manifesto. That is, they claim that biological activity can and does occur *without the presence of any atoms or molecules to which that biological activity can be ascrib*ed.

There exists in contemporary science no paradigm by means of which homeopathy or flower essences can be understood or explained. It is partly for this reason that relatively little attention has been focused upon them in the twentieth century. The absence of a scientific explanation for why homeopathy and flower essences work generates an enormous resistance to any evidence that these preparations have biological activity, either in the human system or in the test tube. More sensitive methods of detecting subtle energies are needed in this new branch of science.

In this book, *essence* refers to the subtle essences that are ingested, including homeopathics, gem elixirs, flower essences, and anthroposophical remedies. Beyond the pages of this book, *essence* is sometimes used to refer to essential oils.

If essences do not contain active molecules responsible for their activity, then how *do* they work? The general idea is that there exists a subtle invisible energy associated with each material substance, like an invisible signature. This energy can be separated or purified away from the material substance and stored in or imprinted upon water. [Unfortunately, mainstream science does not yet have reliable means of detecting such subtle energies.]

Curiously, the notion of essences hovers over the chasm between religion and philosophy on the one hand and science on the other. Major world religions and philosophies have for millennia maintained that there exists within the human frame an immaterial essence that is commonly referred to as the soul or the spirit. The prevalent belief is that this spirit or soul that animates the physical body is capable of surviving the death of the body. This could be described as the vitalistic view of man and of nature. Correspondingly, animals and plants would have their own version of spirit or soul. This principle might explain many phenomena associated with life, as, for example, those elaborated by Rupert Sheldrake,[1] who postulates the existence of organizing energetic fields associated with living systems.

However, the dominant paradigm in biological science has long been the mechanistic philosophy that there is nothing more to life than the chemicals and chemical reactions that occur in the living organism. Based on this paradigm, essences should not, when ingested, affect any biological activity. Moreover, essences have no right to exist at all in this worldview! The entire field of essences is anathema to the dedicated materialist, as is evidenced by the strong emotional reaction to homeopathy that exists in certain scientific environments. However, materialistic science could possibly modify its paradigms to include the notion of a subtle life-force energy without necessarily taking on board the notions of spirit, God, and life after death. Recognition of essences would remove the conflict between science and religion in that science would no longer be contrary to the notion of there being an immaterial spirit or soul. [So although essences currently hover somewhere over the chasm between religion and science, they may in the future form part of a bridge.]

The different types of essences available in the world today are, broadly speaking, homeopathy, tissue salts, flower essences, "environmental" essences, gem elixirs, Aura-Soma, anthroposophical medicine, and "esoteric" essences. It is necessary to understand these types of essences in principle because they form the landscape into which the falling leaf essences are introduced.

Homeopathy

Homeopathy has had a colorful and controversial history since its development by Samuel Hahnemann, a German physician, around the beginning of the nineteenth century. Hahnemann based his new system of medicine on two distinct principles. The first was the law of similars, which held that the medicine used to treat a particular condition should be capable of causing that same condition in a healthy person. (Medicine now, as it did in Hahnemann's time, more commonly proceeds from the law of opposites.) For example, if a person has diarrhea, the physician prescribes a medicine that is constipating in its effect. By contrast, a homeopath would prescribe for diarrhea a medicine that is capable of causing diarrhea in a healthy individual. The second of Hahnemann's principles was that medicine could be greatly diluted without losing its medicinal power. Moreover, the medicine appeared to become, in many instances, more powerful in its action the more diluted it became. Hahnemann used sequential dilutions of medicine (1 part medicine in water to 9 or even 99 parts water) that had been *succussed,* or shaken vigorously, for his treatments.

Although Hahnemann and his followers claimed great cures, his system of remedy preparation was objectionable to the science of both that day and this. The medicinal preparations were diluted to such an extent that their claimed activity seemed unbelievable. Hahnemann himself believed that the dilution could not progress indefinitely without losing effectiveness, but some of his later followers went even further.

Around the beginning of the twentieth century, American physician James Tyler Kent championed the "high potency" school of homeopathy. He and his followers took Hahnemann's process of dilution and succussion to thousands or even millions of repetitions. One of the scales of dilution used in homeopathy is the centesimal scale, abbreviated with a C. A 1C homeopathic preparation is a 1 in 100 dilution of the original tincture. A 3C homeopathic preparation is the result of three successive 1 in 100 dilutions, the total dilution being 1 in $(10^2)^3$ = 1 in 10^6.

Basic chemistry teaches that the number of atoms in a molecule is equal to Avogadro's number, Avogadro's number being 6.023×10^{23}. Therefore, homeopathic potencies beyond 12C (a dilution of 1 in 10^{24}) have *not a single molecule of the original substance* left. Whereas with low-potency homoeopathic preparations (<12C), biological activity might in some way be attributed to the microdose of original substance remaining, beyond 12C dilutions materialistic explanations are impossible. Simple deduction then shows that homeopathy makes the following claim: *Biological activity occurs without the presence of any atoms or molecules to which that biological activity can be ascribed.*

There can be little doubt that homeopathy is effective in practice. It has a worldwide following, including many physicians trained in Western medicine as well as classical homeopaths and naturopaths. One advantage of homeopathy is that there are few if any molecules of original substance present to generate toxicities, side effects, or allergic reactions in the patient. These are significant problems for both pharmacology and herbal medicine. The practicing homeopath takes a comprehensive history and details the person's physical, mental, and emotional symptoms. The most appropriate homeopathic remedy is decided upon from the totality of the person's symptoms, rather than by one or several predominant physical symptoms. Each homeopathic remedy has a detailed symptom picture corresponding to it, which is arrived at by the administration of the substance to many people simultaneously in the homeopathic *proving*, or testing. Most provings were performed in the 1800s, but the results are still invaluable today. There are many branches of homeopathy that have developed over time, and the debate between the purists and those who have developed or extended Hahnemann's ideas continues to rage on.

Before moving on from homeopathy, it is important to note the healing system of Dr. Wilhelm Schuessler, which is based on low potencies of mineral salts. This system is simple and effective and is widely appropriated and understood by the general public. The preparations are sometimes called tissue salts, cell salts,[2] or Schuessler salts. Here, these will be regarded as low-potency homeopathic remedies.

Flower Essences

Dr. Edward Bach was an English physician of the early twentieth century and was well versed in homeopathy. Although seeing great merit in Hahnemann's system of healing, Bach sought a simpler cure that came more directly from nature. His passion to find more effective cures for the health problems confronting him daily led him away from a successful city medical practice to the country.

Bach began to develop flower essences by placing blossoms, leaves, and stems from different flowers in water and letting them sit in the sun. He believed that under the influence of the sun's rays an immaterial essence was transferred from the flowers to the water. The blossoms, leaves, and stems were then removed and the water remaining was considered to be the flower essence.

Bach used his own body as a barometer to sense in detail the mental/emotional state for which each essence was beneficial. He would enter a profound suffering before he actually located the plant from which the essence was to be prepared. In a sense, this physical, mental, and emotional suffering was a revelation of the action of the essence he was about to discover. Bach recorded the symptoms he experienced in detail, and this formed the initial description of the essence. This suffering could be interpreted in several different ways. For example, it could be regarded as a psychic attack from the plant whose essence he was about to extract. In this view, the plant has an intrinsic resistance to its essence being "tamed" or used in human healing. Alternatively, or additionally, the suffering could be regarded as a unification of Bach himself at a spiritual level with the essence of the plant. It has been well known in mysticism for centuries that unification at a spiritual level with another being or essence can generate profound suffering. For example, Christians who have identified strongly with Christ have sometimes experienced the stigmata. Here, the spiritual, psychological, and physical suffering that Christ endured on the Cross is reflected in the body and psyche of the devout. Whatever the explanation of Bach's sufferings and acknowledging that this was perhaps even necessary at that point in time, in general, deducing the action of essences by such personal suffering has little to recommend it! Indeed, Bach himself found this exploration via suffering exhausting and detrimental to his own health.

Thus the Bach flower essences came into being. Mustard, for example, is helpful for deep gloom and depression that descends for no known reason. Sweet Chestnut is needed when a person has reached the despairing final limit of his endurance such that there is only oblivion, suicide, or collapse ahead. Sweet Chestnut can in this situation infuse the person with renewed hope and spiritual vision. Larch is for a kind of brooding despondency that immobilizes or limits a person. When successful, Larch enables the person to shrug off the despondency with renewed enthusiasm and application. Some Bach flower essences are used in combinations. The most famous is Rescue Remedy, which consists of Cherry Plum, Clematis, Impatiens, Rock Rose, and Star of Bethlehem. Rescue Remedy's ability to help in times of crisis has earned it a worldwide reputation with the general public.

Bach's work formed a radical departure from herbal medicine, which extracts bioactive constituents from plants by steeping them in alcohol or very hot water. In contrast, Bach steeped flowers in plain water in the sunlight and then he discarded the plant material. He believed that the water retained a subtle energetic imprint, or essence. Bach's work was also revolutionary in that the flower essences were prescribed based not on the physical symptoms of the patient, but rather on his or her mental/emotional state.

Since Bach's death, his work has been expanded upon by followers. New essences have been created from flowers found around the world, from environments as different as Alaska and Brazil. Many of these are listed in Clare Harvey and Amanda Cochrane's *Encyclopaedia of Flower Essences*.[3]

Environmental Essences

Environmental essences are those drawn from particular features of the environment, rather than from flowers. Any aspect of the environment can potentially be amenable to the development of a corresponding essence. Bach himself pioneered in this area with Rock Water essence, which is drawn from an appropriate pool and is helpful for those who are rigid-minded and self-denying and tend to overwork and overeffort.

A good example of a range of environmental essences, most from Alaska, has been described by Steve Johnson.[4] These include Chalice Well (made in the Chalice Well Gardens of Glastonbury, England, with water from the Chalice Well), Full Moon Reflection, Glacier River, Greenland Icecap, Northern Lights, Polar Ice, Portage Glacier, Rainbow Glacier, Solstice Storm, Solstice Sun, and Tidal Forces. Johnson intuits the action of each essence on the human system by noting the qualities of each environment and the nature of the energies that they express. For example, the essence Solstice Storm is used to cleanse and stabilize the human electrical system. It is believed to be particularly effective in discharging accumulations of static energy held in the body.

Another interesting group in this category are shell essences, developed by Nancy Efraemson and Leonie Hosey in Australia.[5] In their book, *Shell Essences,* they describe twenty-seven different shell essences that address issues ranging from appropriate expression of feelings, spirituality, and group awareness to relationships, femininity, and purification of thought and mind. It might be expected that shell essences bear some similarity to gem elixirs, because the shells are composed of minerals.

Gem Elixirs

Gem elixirs represent another branch of essence therapy.[6] Gem elixirs are prepared by placing an appropriate gem in water and allowing it to sit in the sunlight, where it becomes activated. As with flower essences, some of the essence of the gem transfers into the water over time. Gem elixirs have a significant impact on the physical body; they are both grounding and strengthening. In general, they energize the body, although different gem elixirs benefit different physical problems. They also significantly affect the mental state and assist in the clearing of accumulated stresses. Although gem elixirs are appreciated and widely used by therapists, they are not as well known by the general public as are flower essences.

Aura-Soma

Aura-Soma is another fascinating and well-developed branch of essences, as well as of color therapy.[7] Most essences are colorless to the human eye. Only particularly sensitive people are capable of perceiving their colorful auras, which are also perceptible via Kirlian photography. By contrast, Aura-Soma combines oils and plant extracts into colorful essences that are both unique in their healing qualities and visually appreciated by all. For many people who are skeptical about essences as invisible energies, Aura-Soma provides an excellent entry point into the world of essences. As the saying goes, seeing is believing! The horizontal layering of Aura-Soma bottles with two different colors is artistically splendid.

Aura-Soma came into prominence in the 1980s and 1990s. It was developed by Vicky Wall, who conceived of Aura-Soma during meditation and felt guided to make the first "Balance" bottles without any conscious awareness of their purpose. It became apparent that the colorful variety of essences that make up Aura-Soma had interesting healing properties.

Aura-Soma essences have a greater level of complexity than do flower essences both in their making and in their application. Aura-Soma has won worldwide acceptance among practitioners and their clients. As with Edward Bach, the life of Vicky Wall presents much fine inspiration.

Anthroposophical Medicine

Another fascinating branch of essence therapy is provided by the anthroposophical medicine of Rudolf Steiner (1861–1925).[8] Steiner was an Austrian scholar, mystic, philosopher, and scientist. The striking feature of Steiner was the breadth of his intellect and worldview, which enabled him to make outstanding contributions to education, agriculture, art, dance, metaphysics, and medicine. Anthroposophical medicine has grown out of lectures delivered by Steiner to the medical community from about 1920 onward. The principles underlying anthroposophical medicine are derived from a complex, esoteric worldview that, for the most part, preceded Steiner but of which he was the most eloquent and convincing spokesperson.

Steiner's new system of medicine included not only anthroposophical essences or remedies but also massage, medicinal baths, artwork, and a therapeutic instruction in the art of movement known as eurythmy. Anthroposophical remedies or essences are most closely related to homeopathy in that they are commonly drawn from herbs and minerals and are usually diluted and succussed. Steiner drew upon the Doctrine of Signatures and his own highly developed sense of invisible etheric energies to select and describe remedies appropriate for different conditions.

Manifested Essences

The aforementioned categories of essences are derived from plants, gems, or other aspects of the environment. In that sense, they are all "essences of earth." There exists another, more esoteric branch of essences that those unfamiliar with alchemy might well consider to be nothing more than hocus-pocus or deception. These are manifested essences, which may be thought of as "essences of heaven." *Manifested* in this sense refers to the generation of a subtle energy in the bottle by apparently supernatural means by the conscious intent of the alchemist (the person who is skilled in inventing and preparing essences), without the addition of any extracts or preparations. This process should not be completely foreign to those who work with the earth-based essences; in Aura-Soma, for example, some preparations are enhanced or completed by prayers or invocations as a means of injecting them with more subtle energies.

The Flower Essence Pharmacy (on the Internet at www.flower-essences.com) has a list of esoteric manifested essences that are not made from flora, fauna, or minerals. These include Angelic Essences, Buddha Fire Formulas, Pegasus Starlight Elixirs, Source-Nature-Soul Essences, and White Buffalo Animal Essences.

The notion of manifestation is, of course, far removed from principles of contemporary science. It is already a major paradigm shift to suggest that essences have biological activity without biological molecules to which that activity can be ascribed. It is an even more enormous paradigm shift to suggest that whatever subtle energy these preparations contain can be generated not only from plants and gems but also directly by the trained human mind.

Manifestation of essences is discussed infrequently, perhaps because it is difficult for alchemists and essence practitioners to talk about their work in an era in which they may well be considered mere charlatans. Nevertheless, manifestation works well in *practice*. Two key principles govern the use of manifestation in alchemy. The first is that it is highly inappropriate to seek to manifest an essence that can also be prepared from plants, gems, or other natural sources. That could be construed as simply laziness or ignorance. However, if one wished to construct the aforementioned angelic essences, it would be ridiculous to go out into nature with a butterfly net to catch an angel! In other words, some essences can be extracted or derived from nature and some can't. Only those that can't should be prepared through manifestation. This principle is so obvious that it almost seems unnecessary to state it, yet it is often violated.

The second principle is that manifested essences should be exposed to the scrutiny of one and preferably several other experienced essence workers. There are many who believe they can manifest essences well, but in fact very few can do so reliably and accurately. It is only reasonable that such extraordinary work be evaluated and confirmed by those with the required metaphysical perception.

Are New Essences Needed?

Considering the variety of essences now in existence, including homeopathy, flower essences, environmental essences, gem elixirs, Aura-Soma, and anthroposophical remedies, it is apparent that the twentieth century has brought an explosion in both types and numbers of essences. Perhaps this sudden surge in development has outrun the understanding of essences as a whole.

Accumulating an adequate number of essences in each category is a worthwhile endeavor, but thereafter there are diminishing returns from further essence characterization. Homeopathy, as an example, now boasts more than two thousand remedies. From time to time, provings (testings) of new homeopathic remedies occur, but they raise little excitement. The consensus among homeopaths is that they already have plenty of good homeopathic remedies to choose from for treating the health problems they confront. Indeed, many of the early homeopaths of the nineteenth century restricted their prescribing to ten to fifteen major remedies, with good results. Modern homeopaths often base their practice on one hundred to two hundred remedies that they have come to know very well.

The case is similar for flower essences; the point of saturation or near-saturation has surely been reached. The scope of what flower essences can do is well represented in the many groups of flower essences available from all over the globe.

An important question is whether there is a need for new types of essences or whether the existing categories are sufficient. Historically, it would appear that the need for new essence categories is far from exhausted. The discovery of the new categories of flower essences and Aura-Soma in the twentieth century is generally agreed to have been very important. As the limit of that which is possible with existing types of essences becomes apparent, the search for new essence types begins again.

Perhaps the changing nature of the world contributes to the continuing need for new types of essences. The problems with which individuals, families, and countries grapple most often are quite different from those of a generation or a century ago. Inventors of essences must be in touch with the pulse of society, its directions, aspirations, and inherent problems. Certain types of essences may prove to be effective in one country or culture but quite ineffective in another. Designing essences to fit the needs of different cultures, religions, or world views will be an important aspect of future essence invention.

Essences are called upon not only to treat illnesses but also, increasingly, to assist personal growth or inner transformation. To date, most essence inventors have been medically minded, so that most essences are directed toward the treatment of illness rather than toward personal growth. Essences directed toward personal growth are important not only to facilitate personal and communal evolution, but also to give people better insight and understanding of the illnesses they experience. It may well be that the better path ahead in essence invention is not focused on diagnostic categories of illness, but rather on the beliefs, emotions, attitudes, toxins, and other causal factors that underlie illness in general. In the final estimate, understanding and enabling personal growth and understanding and treating illness with essences may turn out to be one and the same thing.

New categories of essences must meet four criteria to fulfill a worthwhile place within essence therapy.

1. They must be fundamentally different from existing types of essences.
2. They must have a clearly defined purpose or intent that sets them apart from other types of essences.
3. Their importance, distinctive quality, and usefulness must be confirmed by practitioners already familiar with existing essences.
4. The research, development, and preparation of the essences must come up to a professional standard.

New pharmaceutical medications are "proved" by double-blind trials in which patients are given either the medication or a placebo. Neither patient nor doctor knows until after the trial which was medication and which was placebo. There is a tendency to seek to impose this kind of systematic trial upon nonpharmaceutical therapeutic substances, including essences. While I am not opposed to such trials, my opinion is that more weight should be given to the impressions of practitioners with a number of years of experience working with existing types of essences. They can give very good feedback on the value of a new essence. The different levels of subtlety on which essences act make them very difficult to assess with a limited number of objective criteria; they are better assessed subjectively across the full spectrum of human experience. In the case of essences designed to assist personal growth or transformation rather than to treat specific illness, assessment by objective criteria is virtually impossible—there are no symptoms to observe. Subjective feedback from a number of people who have taken such essences is the only yardstick.

The diversity of existing types of essences clearly reflects the needs and thinking of the societies and times in which those types originated. As the twentieth century gives way to the twenty-first, new essences are needed that fit the needs of the fast-paced, technological, intellectual society of today. Yet these essences also need to be deeply rooted in the cycles of the natural world. These new essences must fulfill the four guidelines for new essence types outlined above.

When we ponder either world events or our own lives, we are struck by the way in which the past interweaves with the present in ways that are frequently not constructive. It is often apparent that the conflicts, tensions, misunderstandings, and difficulties of the past, which we thought were long settled or dead and buried, simply resurface in new and, at times, unpredictable ways. Whether we are speaking of our own personal energies, those of families, or even those of nations, there is at times a need to release the energies, issues, and emotions of the past at a more fundamental level than we have done to date. All too often we think that we have dealt with a past issue by a mental decision or by choosing not to think about it any more. Yet it is equally apparent that in our emotional, physical, and even spiritual selves, unresolved aspects of the past lurk in hiding only to reemerge later, often to our frustration, annoyance, and disappointment.

It is to meet [this almost universal need to release the past and cleanse not only the body but also the soul] that I introduce and commend to you the magic of the falling leaf essences.

2 Matching Essence to Need

NO QUESTION IS MORE IMPORTANT in the realm of essences than which type of essence is appropriate for a given situation. A gardener chooses carefully the type of tool he or she employs for different gardening tasks. For digging a trench, a gardener uses a spade. To prune a hedge, a gardener uses pruning shears. We might well laugh at the notion of a gardener hacking away at a hedge with a spade in an attempt to prune it. Although the hedge might well get pruned, the task is made unnecessarily difficult by using the wrong tool, and the end result is that the hedge could be badly hacked and quite unattractive.

Likewise, a golfer selects from his caddy the appropriate golf club for the shot at hand. In considering the choice of iron, the distance to the hole, the wind direction and strength, and even subtler factors such as humidity and psychology may play a role. Similarly, a skilled fisherman considers many factors, including the flow of water in the stream, the weather conditions, the type of fish expected, and the time of day, in selecting which kind of lure or fly to use. In each of these examples, the gardener, the golfer, and the fisherman, a combination of knowledge, observation, and intuition is needed to make an appropriate selection from the array of available tools.

A person using essences generally needs to have several different types of essences in his or her toolbox. It is best stated from the outset that there are many essence practitioners who believe that only one type of tool is needed in the toolbox. There are those who believe, for

17

example, that flower essences are able to meet the full spectrum of humanity's needs. This could be described as the "flower essences are everything" paradigm. Indeed, flower essences have superb areas of strength. As the decades have gone by, however, it has become equally apparent that there are other areas in which flower essences are relatively weak, regardless of how many flower essences one can draw upon from all around the globe. The notion that "flower essences are everything" has ceased to be a paradigm and become instead a syndrome. It generates in its adherents an intense but unfortunate preoccupation with flower essences to the exclusion of any other possibility.

It is quite valid for people using essences to consciously restrict themselves to just one type of essence in order to become highly skilled in its use. This is similar to the situation of a gardener who finds that he or she has a natural affinity or talent for pruning hedges and consequently decides to become a hedge-pruning specialist. We hope that the gardener retains the awareness that although pruning shears are the ideal tool for pruning, other tools are better suited to other gardening tasks. Likewise, homeopaths and flower essence therapists should retain or cultivate the awareness that their fine tools are well suited to some purposes, but there are other essence tools more suitable for other purposes.

My own journey as a full-time practitioner of essences began back in 1987. Having followed up a Ph.D. in biochemistry with six years of post-doctoral work in genetic engineering, I brought to my own use of essences an essentially experimental approach. As a research scientist, one is continually trying different approaches to solving a problem and then critically assessing the results. This is the approach that I brought to healing and which I still use today.

When one approaches healing from this perspective, essences have to earn and justify their place in one's healing toolbox. It is not enough that certain essences have been around a long time and have generally been found to work well. The critical question is how they work in the here and now, when put to the test with actual people with real issues, in one's own experience, year in, year out.

I began back in 1987 with homeopathics and flower essences. Over the succeeding seven years, I came to a profound understanding of the strengths and weaknesses of each of these essence types, through repeated testing of these essences in real-life situations. Even though the results were sufficient to build a busy, seemingly successful practice, by 1992 I became certain that there were alarming deficiencies in my toolbox.

Some of my clients' needs were well met by the essences I possessed, some were partially met, and some were, in my opinion, largely untreated. For the last, I seemed to lack the appropriate tools, and this remained the case regardless of how many different homeopathic remedies I had in my repertoire or how many different flower essences from all around the globe I amassed.

One could perhaps liken healing with essences to the fine sport of archery. When the need presented is very well matched by the essence prescribed, it is a bull's-eye or 10/10 score. When the essence is not quite right but still fairly relevant, the arrow has landed in the first concentric ring, earning a 7/10 score. When the essence approaches irrelevancy to the need or issue at hand, the outer ring of 4/10 or 1/10 is hit, or the arrow might miss the target altogether.

It is noteworthy in this analogy that an arrow that lands even in the outer ring scores something. An oft-repeated misconception among those who use essences is that if the essence "does something," the prescription must have been correct. The archery analogy shows this to be a gross misconception. Even a poorly prescribed essence with only a glancing relevance to the need or issue at hand will generate some movement on some level. Yes, it will score, if only a 4/10 or a 1/10. However, a correct (bull's-eye) essence prescription affords the patient maximum opportunity for effective change or transformation. The closer the appropriateness of the essence for the need, the greater the tendency for change to be permanent rather than temporary. Of course, the actual action of an essence is affected by many factors, including the extent of the person's desire for change, subconscious blockages, and physical vitality. Regardless of these, the potential for transformation in the desired direction is always much greater when the type of essence selected is most relevant and appropriate.

In the final estimate, those who prescribe essences must each decide their own aims and standards. Some will be content to prescribe an essence on the basis that if it "does something," the exercise has been a success. The analogy is archers who are content if their arrow strikes anywhere on the target—at least they haven't missed altogether. Of course, sooner or later an archery coach is likely to consider such students altogether hopeless and give up on them. One would hope that most essence prescribers will not subscribe to this "close enough" philosophy, but instead will want to prescribe the best type of essence in any given scenario.

In both evaluating the action of an essence and making an essence selection, it is important to be very clear as to one's aim. People who want an essence to assist a process of personal transformation, whether self-prescribed or selected by another person, usually have a goal in mind that they verbalize. Sometimes the need is simply to assist a physical problem; at other times it is to resolve an inner or emotional issue. But identifying the relevant aspect or issue to form a basis for essence selection is not as easy as it may first appear. Although the person has voiced a need or issue, body language, intonation of voice, and subtle features of the interaction may suggest an unconscious need or issue that is evident on a more subtle level. Should then the essence prescription be addressed in the direction of the verbalized need or the deeper unspoken need, or both? The answer is that both levels of interaction are generally taken into account. The verbalized need is not all that should be taken into consideration, but it certainly should not be ignored in favor of the unspoken need. In evaluating the subtle interaction, a highly subjective process, prescribers always need to be aware of the possibility that they might be projecting their own needs or emotional intensities onto the client, reading themselves in their client.

The attitude of the person taking an essence is very important in facilitating a favorable outcome. Some people believe that all they have to do is take the essence, and the essence will then fix their problem or issue. Rather more mature and realistic are those who regard the essence as a tool or catalyst that will support a process of transformation that is their own journey and their own responsibility. Those in this second group generally have a much more favorable prognosis, regardless of the need or issue that they present. The action of an essence generally unfolds over a period of time and involves a number of stages. People are quite capable of facilitating or obstructing this process at various stages. They can work either with or against the essence.

The practitioner or prescriber of essences also plays a vital role in the process of transformation that the essence catalyzes. Not only does the prescriber have a responsibility to prescribe an essence of the utmost relevance to the person's need or issue, but he or she is also integrally involved in the flow of energy in the process of transformation. It is absolutely critical that the prescriber of essences has a deep commitment to the process of inner transformation in his or her own life.

Mapping Out the Primary Needs

I use two primary tools in the process of selecting the appropriate type of essence to employ in a given situation. One is the foretuning model, which deals with essence action in terms of four realms, four depths, and four elements. (A book presenting this model will soon be published by Inner Traditions.) This model is strongly recommended to those interested in essences and in natural therapies in general. The other model is expressed in the primary needs chart (diagram 2.1). This is a word-based model that helps explain the variety of needs that people present, and how they relate to the types of essences that are available.

In building up both the foretuning model and the primary needs chart over time, I have drawn on a number of different lines of information and evidence. First, there is the published information about already existing essence types. Second, there is the feedback of my own clients over the years. Third, there is my experience with Thera and Vega machines over the last decade. These bioelectronic machines are invaluable tools both in selecting different essence types and in measuring imbalances that clients present. A word of caution is appropriate here, because theoretically an essence inventor could bias the results with these machines. Inevitably, these machines respond to the energies of both practitioner and client and are not immune to the energetically relayed power of suggestion. Nevertheless, as one of several interactive lines of evidence, these data are extremely interesting and

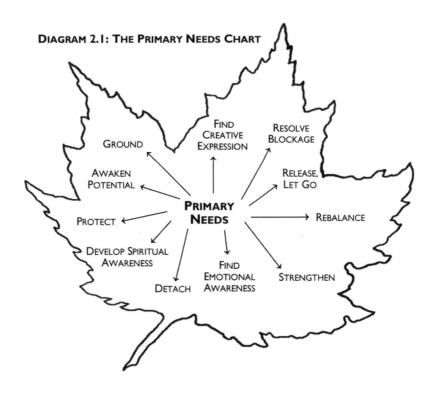

Diagram 2.1: The Primary Needs Chart

GROUND

FIND CREATIVE EXPRESSION

RESOLVE BLOCKAGE

AWAKEN POTENTIAL

RELEASE, LET GO

PRIMARY NEEDS

PROTECT

REBALANCE

DEVELOP SPIRITUAL AWARENESS

FIND EMOTIONAL AWARENESS

STRENGTHEN

DETACH

worthwhile. Fourth, the use of pendulum dowsing has been extremely useful, although subject to similar caution. Fifth, in developing my thinking around essences, it has been invaluable to take time to ponder and reflect. Excessive activity and busyness is of course antidotal to this precious process of reflection.

Perhaps a century or two ago in the Western world, most people seeking medicine or a remedy of some kind simply wanted to feel better. Removal of distressing or painful symptoms was the preoccupation of the physician. Undoubtedly, there is still a demand for the simple desire to feel better, especially in pharmaceutical medicine. However, society has become more complex in so many ways. People are more sophisticated and more lucid in their expression of their needs. It is both very important and intriguing to listen to people express their needs. For what aspect of their life experience do they seek an essence, and why?

Over the years, I have separated the needs people express into the eleven categories of the primary needs chart. It is important to understand clearly the meaning of each category, as these categories will subsequently form the basis for selecting different types of essences.

Strengthen

The need is for some aspect of the person's being, whether physical, mental, emotional, or spiritual, to be made more resilient, to be energized and thereby rendered less susceptible to stress. The need for strengthening clearly implies a present area of weakness.

Rebalance

Sometimes the body's homeostasis, or normal state of activity, is disturbed. The activity of different body organs or systems is adversely affected. When there is a need for rebalancing, the body's endocrine or hormonal system has often been disturbed, as have the immune and/or nervous systems. There is not necessarily a lack of energy, nor is there necessarily a need for strengthening.

Release and Let Go

In this case, the primary need is to detoxify—that is, to clear or resolve something from the system. The release process may pertain to physical toxins stored in the body or to past emotions or issues. More commonly, a process of releasing and letting go of the past is both a physical and a psychological process. In the absence of effective release and letting go of the old, people can find themselves encumbered by the past in such a way as to limit their effectiveness in the present.

Resolve Blockage

Here the need is to clear a fundamental obstruction, which may be spiritual, mental, emotional, or physical in nature.

Find Creative Expression

Here the person observes that some aspect of the flow of energy in his or her daily life is disturbed or interrupted. The need is for an essence or therapy that will restore or enable the creative expression of energy in the relevant aspect of life.

Ground

Many stresses of modern living result in a profound state of imbalance in which a person's energies are unearthed. This is characterized by the inability to think and act clearly, with an undue concentration of energy in the head. Digestion can be impaired, and those afflicted feel "out of themselves" or lightheaded. People in this situation need an essence that rebalances them but also puts them in touch with physical reality. The success of a grounding essence can be ascertained by their ability to perform daily routine tasks from which they previously felt disconnected and by their ability to observe and think clearly about the world around them.

Awaken Potential

The situation arises in a person's experience that he or she feels a need to birth some new aspect of creativity or potential but knows not what or how. There is a definite feeling that it is time to move on to something new or to extend the creative self in a new way. Such a person seeks help in identifying and awakening dormant potential.

Protect

Sometimes people find that they are strongly affected by negativity or other external energies. This is a hypersensitive state of lowered resistance in which they can be reactive to other people's projections or emotional energies, "psychic attack," or even electromagnetic radiation or geomagnetic stress. The impact of these external energies can be so strong and distracting that there is neither energy nor clarity to look at internal issues or other aspects of the situation. The need here is for a specialized kind of strengthening that pertains to the protective layers of the body's aura and the electromagnetic immune system.

Develop Spiritual Awareness

Often, a person seeks insight into the meaning and significance of his or her life circumstances. This is a quest for understanding, purpose, and direction. The person may seek insight from an external person, such as a minister of religion or a clairvoyant. Alternatively, an essence might be prescribed that seeks to cultivate and bring forth the person's own spiritual awareness and insight around his or her circumstances and decisions.

Detach

The situation is created by mental or emotional overinvolvement in a particular scenario or in general. The need is to be able to distance oneself from the relevant stressful situation, as if one were an outside third person. This detachment often gives rise to insight about the situation, in contrast with the previous state of being overwhelmed by it.

Find Emotional Awareness

In a stressful life situation, people's objective in seeking therapy may simply be to become clear as to how they feel. They seek to become more aware of their emotions, which may have been put on hold or suppressed.

To select the appropriate type of essence for a given situation, one first seeks to identify the primary need from the chart. Sometimes there is more than one primary need; in that case, it is important to prioritize the needs expressed or perceived.

Which Essence Type Is Best?

There is no essence type that is very good or even satisfactory in meeting *all* of these many and varied primary needs. In fact, having worked with many types of essences over the past fourteen years, I do not know of any type of essence that addresses more than three of these eleven categories of primary need in a truly satisfactory manner. The oft-repeated claim that a particular essence type, whether homeopathics, flower essences, gem elixirs, or falling leaf essences, can meet all these varied primary needs is, in my experience, patently absurd.

Although no one essence can address all the primary needs, different types of essences work in different ways and lend themselves to addressing different categories of the primary needs. To examine the strengths of different essence types in terms of the primary needs chart, one must take into account the literature around a particular group of essences, as well as one's experience of the essence type in practice over a period of years.

The following represents the distillation of literature, experience, bio-electronic testing, pendulum dowsing, and due reflection.

🌿 Homeopathy

The outstanding asset of this essence type is that it strengthens the entire system. When a person is treated homeopathically, his or her specific problems usually improve, but along with that, a general strengthening takes place. Because of the added strength, the person has greater reserves with which to cope with subsequent life stresses. Homeopathy is also a good system for rebalancing the system as required. Its third strength of note is its ability to promote a release or letting-go process, usually physically but sometimes psychologically, too. This can be seen in the so-called homeopathic aggravation or "healing crisis," in which there is a temporary intensification of symptoms during the releasing and letting-go process.

Reexamining our primary needs chart with homeopathy included (diagram 2.2), we still have a long way to go. Although it is true that homeopathy will have *some* action in other categories, such as in PROTECT or RESOLVE BLOCKAGE, I would rate it no more than 5/10 in effectiveness in these categories. Over time, I have found essences that are so much more effective in the PROTECT and RESOLVE BLOCKAGE categories that I do not even consider using homeopathics in these two areas. Nevertheless, homeopathy excels in the areas in which it is most strong. There is no essence type I am aware of that is more effective in the category STRENGTHEN than homeopathy.

🌿 Flower Essences

In the case of flower essences, we see that in addition to reviewing the literature and using our personal experience as a guide for determining an essence's strength, there is a third guiding principle: the Doctrine of Signatures. Briefly, the Doctrine of Signatures states that we can deduce something about the biological or medicinal action of a natural substance—or its derivatives, such as essences—by

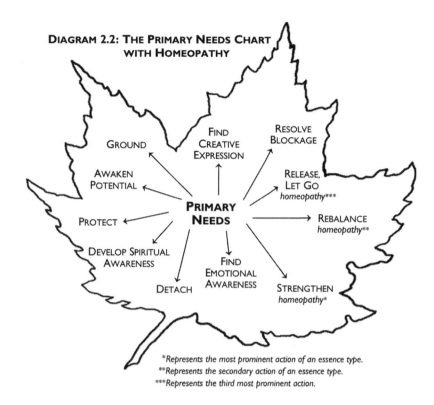

DIAGRAM 2.2: THE PRIMARY NEEDS CHART WITH HOMEOPATHY

GROUND

FIND CREATIVE EXPRESSION

RESOLVE BLOCKAGE

AWAKEN POTENTIAL

RELEASE, LET GO
homeopathy***

PRIMARY NEEDS

PROTECT

REBALANCE
homeopathy**

DEVELOP SPIRITUAL AWARENESS

DETACH

FIND EMOTIONAL AWARENESS

STRENGTHEN
homeopathy*

*Represents the most prominent action of an essence type.
**Represents the secondary action of an essence type.
***Represents the third most prominent action.

observation of its form and function in the natural world.

A flower is an expression of the life force of a plant. The beautiful color, shape, and aroma of a flower speak of the ultimate creative expression of the plant. The Doctrine of Signatures would suggest, then, that flowers and their essences would be of great value in helping people with their creative expression. This deduction is indeed borne out in practice.

In modern science the Doctrine of Signatures is regarded by many as a prescientific notion, such that the above would be regarded as subjective nonsense. However, in alchemy, the Doctrine of Signatures remains just as valid and potent now as it was in the day of Paracelsus.

Observing the response of humans to flowers in general, one notes that flowers are extremely evocative of human emotion. Whether it be tears or laughter or profound nostalgic reflection, the human response to flowers is a common theme both in the media and in real life. Flowers are generally regarded as being important at those key moments in life that are evocative of the deepest human emotions—love, joy, sadness—such as weddings and funerals. This link between flowers and human emotion brings us to the second great strength of flower essences: promoting emotional awareness. A third strength is in promoting spiritual awareness. That is, flower essences help take people out of the humdrum of daily physical existence to give them an elevated or spiritual perspective on their lives and the issues they are working with.

A comparison of the strengths of homeopathy and the flower essences is shown in diagram 2.3. It is very clear that their strengths are quite different. That is, homeopathy is used for strengthening and rebalancing, while flower essences are used for creative expression and emotional awareness. This is perhaps why so many practitioners use both homeopathy and flower essences.

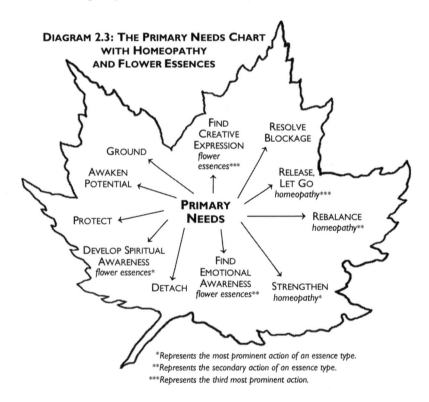

DIAGRAM 2.3: THE PRIMARY NEEDS CHART WITH HOMEOPATHY AND FLOWER ESSENCES

FIND CREATIVE EXPRESSION
flower essences***

RESOLVE BLOCKAGE

GROUND

AWAKEN POTENTIAL

RELEASE, LET GO
homeopathy***

PRIMARY NEEDS

PROTECT

REBALANCE
homeopathy**

DEVELOP SPIRITUAL AWARENESS
flower essences*

FIND EMOTIONAL AWARENESS
flower essences**

DETACH

STRENGTHEN
homeopathy*

*Represents the most prominent action of an essence type.
**Represents the secondary action of an essence type.
***Represents the third most prominent action.

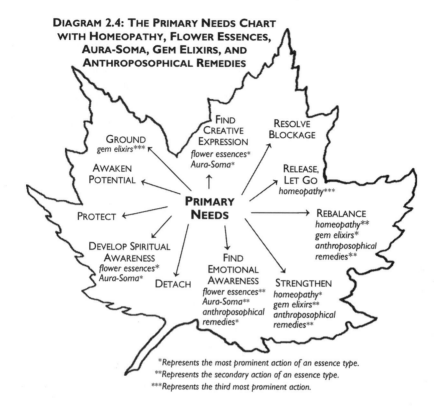

DIAGRAM 2.4: THE PRIMARY NEEDS CHART WITH HOMEOPATHY, FLOWER ESSENCES, AURA-SOMA, GEM ELIXIRS, AND ANTHROPOSOPHICAL REMEDIES

GROUND
gem elixirs***

FIND CREATIVE EXPRESSION
flower essences*
Aura-Soma*

RESOLVE BLOCKAGE

AWAKEN POTENTIAL

RELEASE, LET GO
homeopathy***

PRIMARY NEEDS

PROTECT

REBALANCE
homeopathy**
gem elixirs*
anthroposophical remedies**

DEVELOP SPIRITUAL AWARENESS
flower essences*
Aura-Soma*

DETACH

FIND EMOTIONAL AWARENESS
flower essences**
Aura-Soma**
anthroposophical remedies*

STRENGTHEN
homeopathy*
gem elixirs**
anthroposophical remedies**

*Represents the most prominent action of an essence type.
**Represents the secondary action of an essence type.
***Represents the third most prominent action.

Aura–Soma, Gem Elixirs, and Anthroposophical Remedies

Engaging the same process of reflection around Aura-Soma, gem elixirs, and anthroposophical remedies, we arrive at diagram 2.4. Gem elixirs excel at rebalancing but are also quite useful for strengthening and, to a lesser extent, grounding. Anthroposophical remedies show a pattern similar to homoeopathy in excelling first in strengthening and third in rebalancing. Aura-Soma is very different, with its best action in promoting spiritual and emotional awareness.

Inventing New Tools for the Essence Toolbox

Diagram 2.4 represents my state of awareness toward essences about a decade ago. At that stage, I had many questions but few answers. For people who needed strengthening, rebalancing, creative expression, and emotional and spiritual awareness, I had excellent tools in my toolbox that enabled me to assist them. I also knew that these same tools or essence types were inadequate, ineffective, or even counterproductive when the need was for detachment, awakening potential, protection, resolving blockage, or releasing and letting go.

The overwhelming need presented by many people I have worked with has been to release the old and let go of the past. Sometimes the need is apparently for adaptability, or the ability to change with the circumstances. I tend to think of the need to adapt as simply reflecting the need to release the old and let go of the past, followed by the need to awaken new potential. That is, the "need to adapt" calls forth two primary needs in sequence. People are often unable to move forward in their lives because emotions, problems, and even physical toxins from the past leave them with unresolved issues. From diagram 2.4, it is apparent that homeopathy can help in releasing and letting go. However, I needed an essence type with the *predominant theme* of releasing and letting go. This led me to the development of falling leaf essences, which will be fully described in subsequent chapters. Suffice it to say here that the ability of falling leaf essences to promote emotional, mental, and physical release far exceeds that of homeopathics and, for that matter, flower essences.

Being aware of the lack of adequate tools to meet different primary needs is a powerful catalyst for essence invention. Indeed, once I become aware of a deficiency in the toolbox, a number of people often present with this type of unmet need, as if to impress upon me the urgency of the process of essence invention. Here, we will follow through several examples of the process of essence invention that demonstrate briefly the principles involve (diagram 2.5).

Bark Essences

The primary need category PROTECT expresses a need for protection from some external influence. Some people are much affected by emotions or psychic energies projected from another person or group of people. Some are unduly affected by psychological pressure or by the subtle or overt expectations of others imposed upon them. Some are sensitive to environmental chemicals such as those in car exhaust and perfume fragrances. Others are reactive to electromagnetic radiation or

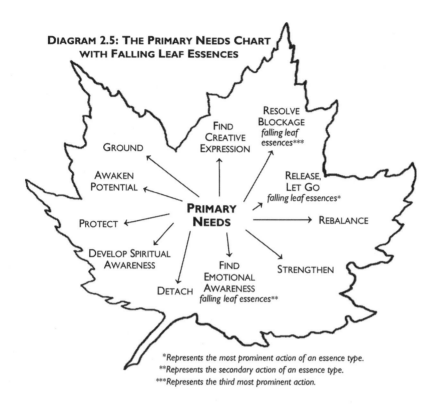

DIAGRAM 2.5: THE PRIMARY NEEDS CHART
WITH FALLING LEAF ESSENCES

RESOLVE
BLOCKAGE
*falling leaf
essences****

FIND
CREATIVE
EXPRESSION

GROUND

AWAKEN
POTENTIAL

RELEASE,
LET GO
falling leaf essences*

PRIMARY
NEEDS

PROTECT   REBALANCE

DEVELOP SPIRITUAL
AWARENESS

FIND
EMOTIONAL   STRENGTHEN
DETACH   AWARENESS
falling leaf essences**

*Represents the most prominent action of an essence type.
**Represents the secondary action of an essence type.
***Represents the third most prominent action.

subtle earth energies that affect their well-being. Obviously, such hyper-sensitive people will derive some benefit from essences that are strengthening. However, what they really need are essences that are protective. Over the years, I tried both homeopathics and flower essences when a protective effect was required. The results were quite limited. For example, I tried the Bach essence Walnut, which claims to be a protective essence against external influences, and the Australian Bush flower essence Fringed Violet, which claims to be for psychic protection. Indeed, they do both have some action in these spheres, yet I would rate them only 4 or 5 out of 10 in effectiveness.

When we return to the Doctrine of Signatures, it becomes immediately apparent that flower essences are a highly inappropriate essence type to address the need for protection. According to the Doctrine of Signatures, the anatomical parts of the plant that play a protective role are likely also to yield protection for human beings. What protects a tree or shrub from the elements and from attack? It is surely the bark, the thick, hard layer that shields and insulates the wood. Therefore, excellent essences for protection can be made from the bark of trees and shrubs.

Imagine that you are out in the woods and are lost. As nightfall approaches, you consider building a hut or protective structure to

---

TABLE 2.1: TWELVE BARK ESSENCES FOR PROTECTION

Tree Name	Description and Primary Action of Essence
Silver Birch	For negativity in close relationships. Recommended in cases where there may be external influences that affect a relationship, perhaps coming from relatives or disapproving friends. For unifying the energy within a household in which tensions and conflicts exist.
Mountain Ash	Assists with protection against "tribal" expectations, such as in the family, when one is expected to enter a particular career because one's father did so, or in a culture, for example, in terms of relationships and marriages. Useful in overcoming fear of public speaking. Protective of the home energetically when used in feng shui.
Tulip Tree	Filters out others' expectations that a person will get an illness— "Your mother had cancer so you will get it, too." Generally applicable when there is a projected expectation of failure from one's own family or a negation of one's path in life.
Golden Elm	Protection from sexual projections in the workplace, a person's social environment, or one's family situation, whether overt sexual advances or the more subtle sexual, energetic projections that often stem from the need to control or take power from another. Also useful for feelings of claustrophobia. Lessens absorption of global or international trauma or emotion. Also protective against cold weather.
Scarlet Oak	Protection from electronic radiation from computers and many other everyday technologies, electromagnetic radiation ley lines and other earth energies, and also subliminal programming. Ideal for those constantly in contact with computers. Also protects against the projection of subservience, wherein technology is the master and we are its slaves. Protective against the ill effects of excessive sun exposure—but certainly not a substitute for common sense.
Pin Oak	Protects against the constant bombardment we face from the overwhelming political, social, and environmental issues on both the national and the international fronts. Offers help for those who find that they are emotionally affected or stressed by all that they see or hear.

Tree Name	Description and Primary Action of Essence
Liquidamber	Offers protection in the workplace from politics and conflicts both seen and unseen. Keeps one from being inappropriately drawn into situations because of emotional attachments. Also protects against political bombardment.
Japanese Maple	Assists in the protection of a person during illness or convalescence. It prevents the ill person from being affected by the expectations and unconscious projections from family and friends. The hypersensitive and weakened person experiences a welcome insulation from the stress both of the immediate environment and of the world at large. A second use of this essence is for a well person who tends to be affected by crowds of people—for example, in a shopping complex or movie theater. In this case, 10 drops per hour, before and during exposure, is recommended.
White Ash	For a person who feels that he has no way out of a situation—he feels imprisoned and that there are no choices to be considered. The classic essence for fear of air travel. Another use of this essence is to protect against unconscious negative projections from the mother.
Canadian Maple	Offers protection from fierce attacks on self-esteem whether they are obvious or subtle energetic projections. Protective against ill effects of hot weather. Also useful in the treatment of agoraphobia.
Scotch Elm	Assists with protection from neighbors or friends and the conflicts that they may seek to draw one into.
Turkey Oak	Filters out the projection of failure that many people endure when others are seeking to keep them within a precast mold.

keep out the wind and cold. Tell me, will you seek to build a hut of bark or a hut of flowers? The question is, of course, ridiculous. We recognize instantly that flowers are not a protective structure. Why, then, do people slavishly insist on using flower essences for the purpose of human protection?

After conceiving of bark essences, I worked with Jennie Richardson and Libby Gordon to develop them, as outlined in table 2.1. I find bark essences satisfactory in meeting a variety of needs for protection, and they have been highly praised by many who have taken them. Bark essences are an example of simple, single-step alchemy. They are each made from the bark of a chosen tree that is floated in springwater for a specified time. Their simple creation, however, does not reflect their powerful application. An essence practitioner who was hypersensitive to the external influences of city life recently wrote to me, saying, "I am really enjoying the bark essences. They do indeed make me feel very protected and nurtured, and it is lovely to feel the forest frequency in the hurly-burly of the city."

Bark essences help people find their boundaries and filter out external influences; they bring clarity, which is often difficult to obtain in our fast-moving, technological society. They also can assist with skin problems and bring metaphysical understanding as to the underlying cause of the skin "dis-ease"—that which gets "under your skin." The intensity of their effect on skin problems is reflected in their order in the chart—that is, Silver Birch first, is appropriate for very mild, recent skin irritation, whereas last, Turkey Oak, would address severe skin imbalances of a chronic nature.

Another suitable group of essences for protection is the shell essences, because these are derived from the external protective skeleton of marine creatures. Otherwise, shell essences show many similarities to gem elixirs, which is hardly surprising given their mineral makeup.

🌱 Seed Essences

Some people seek therapy to help awaken some new aspect of their creative self. Sometimes they identify what it is that needs to be germinated. They are aware that a phase of their life is drawing to a close, and that some new aspect is about to open up and begin, but what, when, why, and how they can't quite say. They sometimes say that they feel "at loose ends" and "unsure of future direction." In such cases flower essences are generally not suitable. Flower essences can take an aspect of the creative self that is already active and enable this creativity to reach its fullness, but they are not well suited for taking creativity that is dormant and inactive and developing it.

Again, we draw upon the Doctrine of Signatures to identify the part of the plant most suited for awakening potential. The notion of awakening implies an initial state of dormancy that then undergoes germination. These words are descriptive of seeds. Seeds have far more creative potential than any other anatomical part of the plant. For example, around my house are many towering mountain ash *(Eucalyptus regnans)* trees. Please note that several different trees have been described as "mountain ash," these bear no botanical relationship to the eucalypt in question. Mountain ash is generally considered to be the tallest flowering tree in the world. Yet the seeds of the mountain ash are very tiny; fifty to a hundred seeds fit comfortably in the palm of one's hand. See what enormous creative potential lies in this tiny seed! Seed essences are supreme among essences when it comes to awakening potential. They gently stimulate the dormant creativity into germination.

Twelve seed essences are described in table 2.2. (There are many more; these twelve simply illustrate the themes and scope of this essence type.) Seed essences act deep within; they arouse dormant creativity from the core of one's soul. Although some essence types such as bark and seed essences can be described to a reasonable extent, one must personally experience the action of seed essences to develop a more personal understanding of them.

TABLE 2.2: TWELVE SEED ESSENCES FOR AWAKENING POTENTIAL

Seed Used	Description and Primary Action of Essence
Aspen	For the normally creative person who has become blocked by an unconscious fear (sometimes almost a paralyzing fear).
Davy Filbert	For the left-brain-dominated person who seeks a fuller expression in life. Helps a person to move out of the dominating mental body and opens up the person to the expression of spirit.
Dove Tree	For people who are frustrated about the lack of creativity in their life, but when they even think of developing some creative expression, become agitated. This essence flows deep into a person's soul and assists with bringing through a deep inner balance and peace.
Glory Vine	For creative people who have become frustrated with their achievements and wish to take their creativity to another level.
Norway Maple	For those who can no longer see any future in their creative expression. Relieves real heart-level despair; assists people in transcending the emotion and allows new hope and energy to flow. Shows them a new pathway in their creative journey.
Pin Oak	Helps people develop and discern a spiritual pathway appropriate to them.
Tulip Tree	Useful for those who have difficulty accepting that we are all creative in our own way, who have an inner anger about other people's creative expression but no belief in their own creativity. Stops a person from comparing her creativity to other people's and encourages her to develop and appreciate her own creativity.
Turkey Oak	A general essence to help release hidden creative potential.

Weeping Katsura Tree	Assists a person who has deep fears of being creative. Brings to consciousness the origins of these fears.
Weeping Willow	Puts one in touch with one's inner childlike imagination. Particularly good for developing creative writing.
White Ash	Assists one in confronting the mental complaints of "I can't" and "I don't have what it takes." Helps remove these blocks to creativity and allows energy to flow again.
Yellow Flowering Currant	Helps a person ground creative ideas and bring them into the physical realm.

✿ Root Essences

When one looks at the theme of grounding, comparing the anatomy of plants and humans is helpful. It is generally regarded in energetic medicine that there are seven chakras, or energy centers, associated with the human being. If we align human anatomy with plant anatomy, we see the correspondence of different anatomical parts of the plant to different chakras or energy centers of the human system. Flower essences are taken from the canopy or crown of the plant and correspond to the three highest chakras—the throat, brow, and crown. From this analogy, we would expect that flower essences would operate mostly in terms of the higher functions—spirituality, the mental/emotional state, and creative expression—and this is indeed borne out by experience.

Based on the anatomical analogy, essences of a plant's root would operate most strongly on the lower chakras—the base (or perineum), the sacrum, and the solar plexus. Root essences are of equal importance to flower essences in alchemy and are the fundamental grounding essences. Because roots radiate into the ground, they draw energy down into the lower chakras, exerting a strong grounding effect. They are ideal to use following the use of a flower essence prescription because they balance the distribution of energy between the chakras.

Root essences are very good for completing transformation initiated by other essences—that is, for getting to the root of the problem. Root essences excel in taking change that has occurred only in the subtle emotional, mental, and spiritual planes and integrating this transformation into the physical body itself. By their very nature, root essences are much more physical in their action than are flower essences, and tend to continue their action until it is completed.

Although I don't advocate the notion, I am often the first guinea pig to try out a new kind of essence. I intuited that the action of the root essence Italian Lavender was to assist with balancing body weight, helping those struggling with extra weight or with anorexia or bulimia. Having wanted to lose about ten pounds for some time, and having had negligible results with other essence types, I was an eager but skeptical guinea pig for this particular trial. I was amazed to see myself shed those ten pounds over the next four weeks. I was also amazed at the intense physicality of the essence, such that my digestive system experienced a fundamental change.

Looking back to the primary needs chart, it is apparent that my weight problem reflected a need for the GROUND category. It was probably an excess of spiritual and emotional development without sufficient grounding activities that led to the weight imbalance. The root essences were the logical essence type to look to for help, and Italian Lavender proved a very effective grounding essence.

The second root essence I experimented with was Happy Wanderer, which is intended to help ease subconscious fears and insecurities. Beforehand, I had assured myself that I had done sufficient work on these issues over time and that this particular root essence would have little effect upon me. It turned out that I was completely mistaken, and for a week I experienced an uncomfortable level of fear and insecurity. It felt as though this emotion was being released from a deep cellular level in the lower half of the body—which corresponds to the base, sacral, and solar plexus chakras. It was a surprise, and it caused me to reflect that many of the earlier approaches I had used to explore these issues had operated mostly on the higher chakras and the central nervous system. That is, the root essence succeeded in excavating fears that other essences around the same theme had not. However, the ease with which Happy Wanderer accomplished its work suggests that other essence types had "loosened" this fear in the lower chakras and made it more readily accessible. The fear was, as it were, ripe for the plucking.

⚘ Transcendence Essence

RELEASE AND LET GO is probably the single most common primary need I've seen presented in my healing practice over the last several years, and it was to answer this need that I developed falling leaf essences.

But a close second would be DETACH. In such cases, people find themselves in a situation in which they are emotionally and psychologically overinvolved. Basically, they are asking not for the situation to be changed but for themselves to have the necessary emotional distance from the situation in order not to be unduly affected. There is, of course, a common myth that feeling detached means not feeling and not caring. Rather, detachment is a position in which one is still aware of, but not overwhelmed by, one's feelings in order that the caring response is optimal. In other words, emotional overinvolvement *reduces* one's capacity to help, and detachment prevents that from happening.

Consider the effect of experiencing a tornado. If one is in the path of the tornado, the experience is indeed terrifying. Even if one physically survives the ordeal, there can be profound, lasting psychological and physical outcomes, such as post-traumatic stress disorder. Imagine, however, that one is watching the tornado from the vantage point of a helicopter five miles away. One can see from the distance the overall situation, and one is less likely to be overwhelmed or paralyzed by fear. Watching the same event ten thousand miles away on an old, small, black-and-white television provides a feeling of even greater detachment. However, with the large screens, graphic color, and realistic sound of modern televisions, traumatic events can now be presented directly in one's living room, as if one were actually present. This makes it difficult to be detached, and one's level of stress can be just as great as if one were at the actual scene. Note here not only that the value of detachment is immense for one's own level of stress and emotion, but that a detached person is generally much more able to be cool and levelheaded in such a crisis and able to help as needed. Being able to back off emotionally from a stressful scene or event is a sign of detachment.

In the present context, *detachment* can be equated with *transcendence*. To encourage detachment or transcendence, we need essences that decrease emotional awareness. One can rule out immediately essence types that have a significant action in increasing emotional awareness. These are apparent from the primary needs chart and include flower essences, Aura-Soma, and falling leaf essences.

The problem is illustrated by considering the ancient four elements of earth, air, fire, and water. Flower essences are made from plant material that grows out of the earth and is composed mostly of water. The water element is associated with the idea of feeling or emotion. The second most important element for detachment is fire. Just as the water element takes us more into feeling involvement with a situation, so the opposing element of fire takes us more away from emotional involvement.

These considerations inspired the development of Transcendence essence, which is a complex essence made in several successive steps (see chapter 6 for details). Note that two of the steps involved in making Transcendence essence involve aeration of the solution (the air element) and exposure to a flame (the fire element). Transcendence essence has a wonderful ability to encourage and enable detachment in even the most difficult and stressful of life circumstances. It has earned great praise over the years from both clients and other practitioners.

⚘ S.A.F.E. Essences

So far, essence invention has been called upon whenever a primary need is inadequately met by existing essence categories. Sometimes, however, one needs to develop a new essence type because the combination of actions an existing essence type offers is undesirable. For example, suppose we want to prescribe an essence for rebalancing. We wish that rebalancing to be as gentle as possible, so we do not want a significant action in certain other categories, particularly RELEASE AND LET GO. The latter sometimes generates turbulence in the short term and can be somewhat demanding. Looking at diagram 2.3, we notice that homeopathy has a significant action in rebalancing, but also in RELEASE AND LET GO. Therefore, it is not well suited to our present intent.

It was for this reason that, in 1992, I developed a new essence category focused on the theme of rebalancing: snow-modified Australian flower essences. Flower essences have their energy concentrated primarily in the spiritual and emotional domains. Snow-modified Australian flower essences are made by placing appropriate flower essences in the snow for several hours. While in the snow, the flower essence goes through a remarkable "death" process, or transformation. After the snow treatment, its energy is predominantly in the physical plane.

This essence type is simply the gentlest rebalancing one I know of, and because it does not encourage detoxification or releasing and letting go, one can prescribe it with confidence in delicate, sensitive situations. Because of the gentleness of these essences, they have for the past decade been my staple prescription for the very young and the very old, and in any situation for which gentle rebalancing support is required. If we abbreviate the name snow-modified Australian flower essences, we arrive at S.A.F.E. The acronymn suits them, I believe, because these essences are, in my experience and in the experience of several other practitioners, very safe. I would not suggest that homeopathic remedies are *unsafe*, but their propensity to cause a "homeopathic aggravation" or "healing crisis" makes prescription in delicate situations a real test of skill for experienced homeopathic practitioners. Snow-modified Australian flower essences, by contrast, are relatively easy to learn and to use, though they must still be prescribed with care.

As shown by the abbreviated listing given in table 2.3, each snow-modified Australian flower essence pertains to a particular organ of the body. (A more detailed listing is available on our Web site: www.advancedalchemy.com.au) These essences are homeostatic—that is, they modulate organ activity back toward normal. If the organ is over-active, the essence operates to lower activity toward normal. If the organ is underactive, the essence operates to raise activity toward normal.

TABLE 2.3: TWELVE SNOW-MODIFIED AUSTRALIAN FLOWER ESSENCES FOR REBALANCING

Organ/System of Primary Action	Flower
Arteries	*Zieria species Q*
Brain	Hairy Guinea Flower
Breasts	Sticky Boronia
Eyes	Yellow Buttons
Heart	Native Violet
Immune System	Sidney Rock Rose
Kidneys	*Hibbertia cistiflora*
Liver	*Persoonia nutans*
Lungs	Yellow Emu-Bush
Lymphatic System	*Phebalium squamulosum* ssp. *ozothamnoides*
Muscles	Blue Lechenaultia
Central Nervous System	Fringed Heath Myrtle

Essences in Practice

The material in this chapter leads one to the golden rule in essence therapy: Always use the essence type that is most appropriate for the problem at hand. For example, if the need is PROTECT, the bark essences are supreme. If the need is FIND CREATIVE EXPRESSION, flower essences are excellent. If the need is GROUND, root essences will excel. If the correct *type* of essence is prescribed, good results are usually forthcoming, even if the particular essence(s) prescribed is/are suboptimal. This is because, for example, in the case of protection, all bark essences have a generic protective effect, as well as excelling in their particular aspect of protection. All root essences encourage the process of grounding, even if they are not exactly the right ones for the case in hand.

I would not suggest that choosing essences within categories or types is unimportant or to be taken lightly. Rather, I strongly remind the reader that getting the essence type right is fundamental and of the utmost importance. If you are trying to use seed essences for the purpose of protection or flower essences to encourage grounding, or any

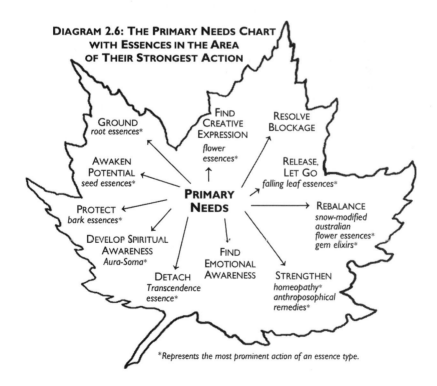

DIAGRAM 2.6: THE PRIMARY NEEDS CHART
WITH ESSENCES IN THE AREA
OF THEIR STRONGEST ACTION

GROUND
root essences*

FIND
CREATIVE
EXPRESSION
flower
essences*

RESOLVE
BLOCKAGE

AWAKEN
POTENTIAL
seed essences*

RELEASE,
LET GO
falling leaf essences*

PRIMARY
NEEDS

PROTECT
bark essences*

REBALANCE
snow-modified
australian
flower essences*
gem elixirs*

DEVELOP SPIRITUAL
AWARENESS
Aura-Soma*

DETACH
Transcendence
essence*

FIND
EMOTIONAL
AWARENESS

STRENGTHEN
homeopathy*
anthroposophical
remedies*

*Represents the most prominent action of an essence type.

other inappropriate combination of essence type and need, you have set yourself up for failure from the outset. Even the best and most careful prescribing from within an appropriate group of essences can at best give a very modest and dampened outcome. A ready reckoner of suitable essence types for different primary needs is shown in diagram 2.6.

✽ Adapting the Chart to Fit Your Needs

As time goes by, the needs addressed in essence therapy change to some extent. One is tempted to add to or subtract new and old categories of need from the chart. For example, in recent times I have thought of adding a new category, ADAPT, to the chart. I see a growing number of people express a need in terms of their inability to change at a rate equal to that of the external world around them. In other words, they feel overwhelmed by change and feel unable to keep up with it. While their feelings may contain elements of a need for detachment or even release and letting go, they are actually asking for something different and more than these categories supply or enable. They are asking for their ability to adapt to change or increase. Falling leaf essences excel in this category. The reason I have not added ADAPT to the chart is that, as previously stated, I believe this need is basically a combination of two existing categories in sequence—that is, the need to release and let go, followed by the need to develop new potential. Falling leaf essences first, followed by seed essences later, facilitate this vital process of adaptation. So when I use the term *adapt*, it calls to mind first the falling leaf essences, but it also has a reminder that something else, probably a seed essence, might be required subsequently to open up new possibilities and directions. Clearly, if we follow the theme of releasing the past and letting go of the old to a ridiculous extreme, we end up having let go of everything and having nothing at all left in our lives!

Another possible category of need emerging in recent times is INCREASE EMPATHY. There are several essence types that can increase emotional awareness, but in this case personal emotional awareness constitutes part of the problem. People very rarely will state that they are excessively self-absorbed or preoccupied with their own issues and emotions, yet this increasingly appears to be the case in recent times. Lack of empathy is a possible downside to our modern era of personal growth and inner transformation. When people become preoccupied with the issues and emotions they are dealing with, sometimes the focus becomes *my* feelings, *my* issues, *my* purpose, and *my* life, to the exclusion of a real feeling of involvement with the world around them.

Their need is partly for detachment but also for a greater ability to feel into the emotions and issues of other people. Often, all that is needed for healing to occur is a shift in focus from a preoccupation with self to a feeling of involvement in the bigger picture. One's problems take a different and much more manageable perspective when one sees the value of one's relationship to other people and the world. Bark essences are quite good for this purpose, because the bark represents that outer layer of connection between the tree and the external world. However, if this need presents more strongly, I may in the future seek an essence type very specifically designed to address this need.

In this chapter, a simple model has been presented that expresses different types of needs and relates those needs to the essences that are best suited for addressing them. The approach is neither more nor less than basic common sense. But the primary needs chart is essentially dynamic. For potential or present essence practitioners, it is useful to consider these vital questions:

What type of needs or issues present in the people I work with?

Which of these needs are adequately met by the essence type(s) and other modalities that I use?

Where are the gaps between the needs I see and the essences or other modalities that I use? Do these gaps call for new tools?

In considering these questions, you the reader may come up with a primary needs chart that looks quite different and uses different words from my own. Obviously not all will agree with the primary needs that I have presented. The needs of your clients might be somewhat different from those of mine. The results you have had working with essence types may be different from my own. In the final estimate, the primary needs chart is simply a dynamic means of associating need and essence type rather than a divine infallible edict.

℘ Intuition versus Logic

A major concern is the near vacuum in thinking about essence prescription that seems prevalent in many circles today. The remarkable notion exists that one can use essences intuitively, without engaging the mental faculties at all. Indeed, two therapists refused to attend a seminar I conducted on essences but still wanted to purchase some essences. Their reason for avoiding the seminar was that they could do without "all that mind stuff." The vehemence with which that phrase was expressed conjured in my mind an image of a vat of poison! Indeed, there exists a curious polarization in healing wherein conventional Western medicine excels in the rational, logical process but somewhat downgrades or disrespects the intuitive or spiritual aspects. Conversely, many alternative practitioners are well developed intuitively and spiritually but the rational, logical process is anathema to them. My own position is fairly simple: We need both the rational/logical and the intuitive/spiritual in balance and harmony to enrich each other in the learning process.

⁂ Using Essences in Balance

Most essence types begin to have detrimental effects if taken for too long. This appears not to be the case with homeopathy, where there is such an enormous diversity of types of substances used and different strengths and potencies. But it is still possible to overdo homeopathic treatment. Taking a number of flower essences in succession over months or even years isn't a particularly good idea. Overconsumption of flower essences could, over time, overconcentrate energy into the higher chakras, resulting in spiritual/psychological development and growth but at the expense of the energetics of the lower chakras. This, in turn, can result in sluggish digestion and elimination, lowered libido or sexual interest, and a partially ungrounded state.

Root essences could rebalance the state that overconsumption of flower essences would lead to, but a prescription of too many root essences in succession is not a good idea either. It could lead to an overconcentration of energy in the lower chakras and even an inflammation of parts of the lower body, due to excessive physical change without sufficient time for integration.

In my own healing practice, the issue of too many prescriptions of one type of essence seldom if ever arises. This is because the primary need of clients tends to change from visit to visit, and therefore the essence type changes as well. For example, a person might present with an overwhelming need to release and let go of a particular issue or past event or emotion. The first prescription corresponding to the need is surely falling leaf essences. Several weeks later, after speaking with the client, it is apparent that there is much less intensity around the original issue or emotion; the releasing and letting-go process has been reasonably effective. Yet now I have the impression that the releasing and letting-go process has been quite demanding, and that the person is somewhat depleted and out of balance. So the primary needs now are STRENGTHEN and REBALANCE. Now I may switch to homeopathy or perhaps gem elixirs. Several weeks later, the person is feeling pretty good but seems unsure as to future plans or directions. The primary need has again shifted, this time to AWAKEN POTENTIAL, and therefore seed essences might be used. If this person comes back later, enthusiastic about some new project or venture but with energies somewhat ungrounded, root essences might follow.

There are, of course, many different directions that the above scenario could take. In my experience, it is rare to use the same type of essence more than twice in succession. One should also be aware that essences are potent catalysts of change, and that people often need a break from them. That is, sometimes so much change has been stimulated that several months without essences serves the need for them to integrate the changes and observe how their life has altered as a result, rather than plunging ill prepared into further change. Personal growth and development can become an addiction just as destructive as drugs or alcohol if the person's body and being are not allowed time to integrate change. A common modern delusion is that personal growth or inner change can be fast-tracked, such that we will arrive next year at an enlightened state of being where all is love and light! Rather, personal growth requires years and even decades of patient application to produce enduring results.

Commitment to Inner Growth

Essences not only are important for healing physical and psychological illness and imbalance, but also are invaluable tools for personal growth and inner transformation. The need for inner transformation as well as physical well-being seems overwhelming as we enter the twenty-first century. It is clear that there exists an enormous commitment to ongoing technological advancement in Western nations in particular. Unless this is matched by a high level of commitment to inner, spiritual, emotional, and psychological transformation, the outcome is almost entirely predictable. The growing chasm between technological advancement and inner growth generates a disparity increasingly manifest in destruction. Essences are one means by which the chasm can be addressed.

Finally, this work introduces falling leaf essences as a fundamental essence type equally important to flower essences and other essence categories. These falling leaf essences excel in their areas of strength, letting go of old emotions, issues and beliefs, as well as accompanying physical toxins. They are also excellent for emotional awareness. However, please note that they are contraindicated for other purposes, such as strengthening, balancing, and detaching. Somehow, many people become so enthusiastic about a new essence type that they seek to sprinkle it over all of humanity in order to cure all problems! In their enthusiasm, they forget about balance and about using each type of essence only in its areas of strength. It cannot be overemphasized that the extent of benefit that humanity derives from falling leaf essences and other essence types depends entirely on the wisdom and discernment around their employment in the healing process.

3 Release and Let Go: The Primary Need of the Twenty-First Century

ADVANCES IN ESSENCE THERAPY ALWAYS OCCUR within a cultural context. Indeed, one might argue that the conditions in a culture call forth essence invention. For example, the depressed conditions of England in the early twentieth century encouraged Edward Bach to invent flower essences. These essences helped to "brighten up" people, enabling them to have a fresh outlook on their lives in the midst of trying times. As the twentieth century progressed and became more sophisticated, a more sophisticated system of essences was born in Aura-Soma. These and other essences retain their vitality at the present time.

As the twentieth century gives way to the twenty-first, humanity individually and collectively faces enormous challenges. One major constellation of stressors arises from the pace and extent of change that people face in their lives. Areas as diverse as personal relationships, housing, transport, telecommunications, technology, leisure pursuits, clothing, and the nature and environment of work are all rapidly changing. A significant new industry has developed to help people cope with change—"personal change consultants" or "institutional change consultants," comprising counselors, psychologists, and a range of other therapists. Ironically, many of these personal change consultants are themselves struggling to cope with the extent of change in their own lives. Sociologist Alvin Toffler has made a strong case for the argument that change occurring simultaneously in many different aspects of people's lives will overwhelm them.[1] Inherent in this work is a realization of the dangers posed by increasing rates of change in society.

A noteworthy feature of many of these changes is that people often have little if any choice about experiencing them. For example, technological change is rampant, and an employee faced with the introduction of computerized systems has no choice but to adapt. As countries and institutions change, change is enforced on individuals and families. This absence of choice about change generates in individuals and even communities a feeling of powerlessness that can make such change distressing.

The human being has an impressive resilience in the face of change. People generally handle significant change in one area of life. A worker might, for example, successfully negotiate the stress of the introduction of computerized systems. This same person might be capable of enduring the stress and grief of breakdown of an intimate relationship or death of a loved one. This person might also be able to negotiate the stress of a learning or behavioral difficulty in his or her child. However, when these stresses are mounted on top of one another, the ability to adapt can be overwhelmed. In this case, physical or psychological symptoms arise. These psychological symptoms can take on a number of forms, from despair, depression, confusion, and disorientation to rage and psychotic behavior. The physical symptoms can be varied and may not be apparently associated with the earlier stresses. Medicine has in recent times identified post-traumatic stress disorder. In this syndrome a variety of physical and psychological symptoms are generated after an identifiable trauma of some kind. More subtle but perhaps even more common is the generation of a similar symptom picture to that of post-traumatic stress disorder not by one trauma but by the accumulated stress of many changes over an extended period of time. It is, of course, entirely impossible to prove that the cause of such an illness is the accumulated stress of change, although that often represents a sensible conclusion.

Our Changing Minds

Change is capable of generating superficial or profound stress in the mental realm. The notion of superficial stress is illustrated by rearranging the furniture in one's living room. One will almost certainly go to sit down where the familiar chair used to be. Here, awareness lags behind reality, and this incongruence generates a temporary mental stress. In the mental realm, habitual patterns take time to change, and this change generates a superficial stress. The notion of profound stress is illustrated by rearranging the furniture and replacing one's normal chair with a new reclining leather chair. This chair is beautiful and luxurious; its opulent comfort and lavish appointment make it unlike any chair one has owned in the past. Suppose that the idea of owning such an ostentatious, extravagant chair challenges one's basic self-concept that was formed decades ago in childhood; this could generate a profound stress. That is, in order for one to sit in that chair regularly and not feel uncomfortable or stressed about it, something fundamental about oneself needs to change.

Base-level mental programming, which is instilled during childhood, can be difficult and time-consuming to change. This remains true despite the claims of numerous therapies and short courses that offer a neatly packaged overnight enlightenment. For example, those who grew up in the Great Depression of the 1930s and then experienced the frugality enforced by World War II might lead lives today as if they were still in poverty. The current reality might be that they are actually quite affluent. Clinging to outmoded notions of scarcity, they have not adapted adequately to new circumstances.

When confronting a change to base-level mental programming, the almost universal reaction is fear. To change a fundamental aspect of oneself is, in a sense, a death experience—a long step beyond safety and security. That fundamental aspect has become part of one's identity, and the very notion of changing it activates the self-preservation instinct. One's mental realm—identity, memories, observation, and so on—is, of course, inextricably linked with one's emotional realm; change in the mental realm is always accompanied by emotional change, and vice versa. But change in the emotional realm can be even more demanding and time-consuming than it is in the mental realm. For example, one may have accepted in the mental realm that a loved one had passed away years ago but at times still be troubled emotionally about it. The emotional realm is still adjusting to a trauma that occurred years ago.

Life in modern environments with high levels of water, food, and air pollution generates the need for change in the physical realm—that is, for detoxifying the body on an ongoing basis. This has given rise to branches of therapy such as clinical ecology and aspects of naturopathy. But as with emotional and mental change, the need for physical change should not be considered in isolation. Physical toxins can represent suppressed emotions or obsolete mental programming, such that physical detoxification can benefit mental and emotional realities.

One also perceives that high rates of change lead to an incongruity among different levels of human experience. Generally speaking, people can change their mind about something much faster than they can change their emotions or their bodily reaction. For example, if I live in a racist society, I might decide mentally that racism is bad and I want nothing to do with it. However, if I have not released ancestral beliefs and programming about racism, my own emotions about it, and whatever racist energies I have absorbed from the culture in which I live, racism might still be an integral part of my energies, or who I am. It is a gross misconception to believe that just because we have made a mental decision about something, all the other levels of our being have spontaneously and immediately adjusted to this mental decision. This incongruity can often be seen quite visibly. One may listen to people speaking about themselves and conclude that what they are saying does not correspond to the energy they project or to their body language. Such an incongruity often indicates that the speaker needs to release and let go of certain old realities, programming, beliefs, perceptions, and emotions.

Releasing the Past

Whereas the spiritual quest of peoples of past generations was for enlightenment, self-realization, or simply happiness, in today's rapidly changing world the cry is for adaptability—the ability to survive and adjust functionally to change.

Thus, if one were to express the need of our times in terms of essences, it would be for a group of essences to help release the old and let go of the past, spiritually, mentally, emotionally, and physically. Such a group of essences would significantly contribute to our ability to cope with the overwhelming rate of change we see in our lives.

🍂 Nonessence Therapies

It is noteworthy that a number of nonessence therapies have come into being that answer this need. For example, Phyllis Krystal's book *Cutting the Ties That Bind* has proved immensely useful to those wanting to dissociate from aspects of the past.[2] Krystal describes a simple, visual, ritual process by means of which one can dissociate from a person, issue, or emotion of the past, so that the connection is no longer functional. Likewise, much of the work of the modern-day army of counselors and psychologists has to do with helping people come to terms with events from the past and thereby relieve adverse effects on the present.

Therapies that deal with issues of the past as obstacles to positive change in the present are not without their inherent potential problems. Any therapy that tackles past issues will tend to cause a temporary concentration of awareness in the past. This becomes a real problem when the person is unable to return his or her focus in due course to the present. For example, through counseling, an employee comes to understand that his concealed rage toward his boss has to do with unresolved and unrecognized anger toward his father. As this suppressed emotion is released, he may have flashbacks to different incidents from the past, perhaps when he was beaten or ignored by his father. This turning of attention to the past, emotionally and mentally, may be necessary during the period of therapy. But when therapy is effective, what then follows is a significant period of time in which the person reports a greater ability to be fully present in the here and now. In this example, one would also look for the employee to have much less concealed emotion toward his boss.

However, it is unfortunately true that therapy tackling issues of the past often fails because it never adequately reconnects to the present.

The purpose and point of such therapy is surely to help people cope with their present lives and changes therein. Yet people who begin to look at their past often open a Pandora's box that then requires years or even decades of seemingly endless sorting out. Such people are perpetually "in therapy," and their awareness becomes permanently centered in the past, often in their childhood years. They seek to "clear everything" from their past and thereby reach some mythical future enlightenment and happiness. Their lives in the present often lose all momentum, their relationships with people often decline, and they become much more introverted and self-centered. One sees this pattern repeated with regularity. Such adverse consequences of therapy must surely be attributed at least in part to therapists who cling to their clients long after the original need to resurrect the past has been met. In addition, with clients who reenter the past on a permanent basis via therapy, one must suspect a powerful subconscious sabotage pattern in operation. The key is to do just enough work on the past to enable effective change in the present, then to refocus on the present.

🕮 Finding the Answer in Nature

In order to find a group of essences that particularly relate to releasing the old and letting go of the past, it is necessary to study nature. That is, one must observe and reflect upon nature and the patterns of change inherent therein. Of course, this is patently obvious, because all essences are ultimately or directly derived from nature.

Change is the one constant that can be observed in nature. Wherever around the world one is, change is happening—sunrise, sunset, the migration of birds, the movement of the tides, the formation of ice, the melting of ice. Much of this change is cyclical in nature rather than purely random. For example, every day there is both sunrise and sunset. Every high tide is followed by a low tide. Cycles such as these may be observed within a single day. More prolonged observation of nature reveals cycles that are of longer duration. With the exception of the equatorial and polar regions, the rest of the globe experiences to a perceptible extent the four seasons of spring, summer, autumn, and winter.

The four seasons profoundly influence the cycles of plant life. Spring is the season of explosive growth. In the plant kingdom, seeds germinate

to bring forth vigorous shoots. Many established plants begin to produce new growth, including flower buds. Summer is the time when the
sunlight is both strongest and longest; it is the season of full bloom,
when flowers are produced in the greatest array. Autumn is the season
of shedding or releasing that which is deteriorating. Many deciduous
trees shed their leaves altogether. Flowers wither; annual plants die. Winter is the season of cold. Plants that are capable of surviving the winter
are in survival mode. The hardy seeds of plants lie dormant, waiting for
spring.

It's important to note that the four seasons are interdependent.
Clearly, it would be impossible to have a spring with lots of new, explosive growth unless there had been a prior autumn in which much old
plant material had been shed and composted. Likewise, summer
requires a prior winter's dormancy and spring's melt.

On a human level, summer is overwhelmingly popular. Holiday des-
tinations are generally sold to the public based on promises of sun and
warmth, not cold and dampness. Our homes are artificial indoor environments intended to make available the light and warmth of summer
all year round. Decorative bouquets are made of flowers in full bloom,
not of spring buds, winter seeds, or fallen leaves of autumn. As soon as
there is any sign of decay in such a bouquet, the offending flower
heads are promptly removed. Likewise, fruit and vegetables in super-
markets must be summer-perfect, free of any blemish or fault. There is
a notion of youth and perfection that pervades the idea of summer
that we hold in our consciousness. Summer forms an essential aspect
of contemporary mythologies of happiness. The hero in a Western
movie rides away into the sunset, not into a rainstorm or blizzard. In
the "happily ever after" endings to movies, the weather is most often
pristine summer in all its glory. Psychologically, summer, with its light
and warmth, is associated with feelings of hope, optimism, and energy.
In contrast, winter, with its dimmer light and cold, is associated with
feelings of depression, lack of motivation, and bleakness—in short, the
"winter blues."

In Western cultures there exists a profound separation between people and nature. People exist in a state of perpetual summer. Their
houses, workplaces, and cars are heated and air-conditioned to ensure

balmy summer temperatures all year round. They may observe the sky-line through windows, but what they see out there, be it rain, hail, or shine, is of purely academic interest; it has little if any actual effect on their lives. They do not need the rains for crops or for drinking or cooking water. Even the modern diet exists almost independently of the seasons. Whereas in times past, particular foods were available only when they were in season, now they are produced year-round in artificial environments or flown in, if necessary, from a distant part of the country or world.

Complementing the overwhelming popularity of summer is a lack of ease with autumn and winter. This is perhaps partly because these seasons are a reminder that nothing in the material realm is permanent, that even the magnificent blooms of summer are ephemeral. It was the sadness and grief associated with the realization of impermanence in the material world that motivated the Buddha thousands of years ago to attain a detachment from the world and suffering. Also, spring and summer are generally seasons of high energy, whereas autumn and winter are seasons of reduced energy, or energy that is turned inward rather than outward. Winter takes one into oneself; it is a time of introspection and self-knowing. For many, this is not a pleasant experience; it is one they would prefer to avoid by perpetuating summer.

We can compare the four seasons, and the human discomfort with autumn and winter, to Western cultures' treatment of the human existence. Spring could be considered the years from birth to twenty; summer, the years from twenty to forty; autumn, the years from forty to sixty; and winter, the years from sixty onward. Glamorous models in magazines and on television are exclusively in their mid-thirties or younger, corresponding to summer. There are no seventy-year-old supermodels. As the autumn of human experience progresses, individuals who begin to suffer from decreased mental or physical ability are frequently placed in nursing homes, where they are hidden from the view of the public. Death is usually concealed, occurring in hospital beds or nursing homes, with the bodies of the deceased whisked away under covering sheets.

An enormous industry exists around the perpetuation of the appearance of the summer season of life in the physical realm. Anti-aging skin preparations, diets, supplements, and cosmetics abound, along with cosmetic surgery. With this perpetuation of the illusion of youth (for those who can afford it), there is a basic underlying premise that aging is undesirable and to be avoided whenever possible. In Western cultures, there is little notion of grace, dignity, and beauty in aging.

Bearing in mind that the types of essences developed in a society will represent the perceptions and attitudes prevalent in that society, it is understandable why some common essence types are based on summer. This is the case with flower essences. The exclusive dependence on flower essences is clearly symptomatic of a cultural belief in the all-sufficiency of summer. Why look to other seasons when summer is so wonderful! People want the energies of summer and desire to remain in a state of maximum energy, maximum creativity, and maximum abundance all the time.

The pattern depicted by Western society is to cling desperately to summer in a vain effort to perpetuate this season indefinitely. This is ultimately impossible, yet even the stubborn clinging to summer and the refusal to release and let go occur at a high price. This price is paid on many levels in society, ranging from effects on individuals to problems that grip whole societies. Whenever we refuse to release and let go when appropriate, we accumulate an unnatural toxicity at some level of our being. Such unnatural toxicities act like latent malignancies in the soul, the body, and the fabric of society at large.

On the level of the individual, the failure to release and let go takes its toll both psychologically and physically. For example, emotional toxicities resulting from a failure to release and let go can ultimately present in psychosis and a range of other psychological and psychiatric disorders. Indeed, it is doubtful that we can even maintain a basic level of sanity without effective processes of releasing and letting go operating in both our psychological and our physical domains. On the physical plane, emotional suppressions such as may occur with guilt, grief, and anger contribute to serious illness including heart disease and cancer.

Even more insidious, however, is the toll that the failure to release and let go takes on society at large, unrecognized. For example, young people who do not learn how to release and let go on the emotional sphere of life can accumulate emotional toxicities that cause them severe emotional pain. In order to relieve this pain, they then turn to drugs. In order to support their drug habit they turn to crime. Alternatively, people who have both severe emotional and psychological toxicities can become vulnerable to extremist views and extremist actions. After all, the unnatural toxicities resulting from a failure to release and let go can become extreme and then result in extreme action. Such unnatural toxicities of the soul and mind can distort a person's judgment and make them vulnerable to manipulation by others. Indeed, one could develop from accumulated mental and emotional toxicities a plausible hypothesis for the generation of evil in the world.

The beauty of the falling leaf essences extends far beyond the immediate action of these essences. Over time they actually teach us how to release and let go in a graceful and natural manner without undue stress. They powerfully encourage us to move through the seasons of life in a flowing manner. Our first response to the need to release and let go is often fear. Indeed, it is fear that holds back the Western world from the autumn season and its falling leaf essences. Yet when we contemplate the consequences of not releasing and letting go, of stagnation, suppression, toxicity, and clinging to outmoded things, we recognize that this is a far more fearful reality to enter! In the courageous moment in which we make the decision to "release and let go," we avert multiplied suffering in the future.

It is interesting to note that some cultures have a particular aversion to "releasing the old and letting go of the past." Here in Australia, for example, much of the approach to life can be summed up in the oft-repeated Australian phrase "She'll be right, mate." The meaning of this phrase is an optimistic confidence that if you leave things alone, they will work out of their own accord. You don't have to worry about anything. If you find a problem, simply ignore it and it will go away or sort itself out! If something from the past bothers you, just forget about it, "She'll be right, mate!" A little reflection upon the meaning of this phrase reveals a life philosophy that is exactly the opposite of the understanding we have developed around the falling leaf essences. People do not see the need to release the old and let go of the past. By contrast, my own belief is that unless the past is dealt with, it tends to resurface in ugly and unwanted ways.

An interesting view around essence invention is that essences come into being in a geographical location where they are needed most. For example, in the depressed conditions in England in his day, Dr. Bach's flower essences were needed to "brighten" people up, to give them the optimism and energy of the summer season. In my perception, falling leaf essences are greatly needed in Australia in order to facilitate the release and letting go of aspects of the nation's past that prevent progress on many levels. For example, it is perhaps long past time for Australia to move from being a British colony to becoming a republic, an independent nation. The present leadership of Australia doesn't think so. Likewise, the shocking abuse that the Aboriginal people of Australia suffered under white settlement perhaps calls for a national apology by the Australian government to the Aboriginal people for the deeds of our white ancestors. This would perhaps form a vital link in a healing process. The present leadership of Australia doesn't think so.

The Birth of Falling Leaf Essences

The notion of falling leaf essences first occurred to me during a trip to Bright, in northern Victoria, Australia, in the autumn of 1994. The old adage states that there is nothing new under the sun. Surely sometime, somewhere, someone has floated falling leaves of autumn in water and prepared essences from them before now. But I had never heard of them.

Bright is a historical town about a four hours' drive northeast of Melbourne. It built up rapidly in the 1850s in the era of the gold rush. It is world renowned for the autumn colors of the deciduous trees that line its streets and avenues. I had traveled to Bright for a week's vacation by myself. I had great expectations for plenty of walking and fresh air and, perhaps, a sense that some new phase in my life was about to unfold. I had been working as a therapist with homeopathy, flower essences, gem elixirs, and nutrition for about seven years. Although there are always new possibilities of working with these fine tools, I felt basically as though I had come to the end of an apprenticeship and something new was about to be birthed.

During my time in Bright I indeed walked for several hours each day. The mountain air was crisp, and the variegated autumn leaves were thick on the ground and continuing to fall. Surprisingly, the more I walked in this environment, the more energy I gained. The air seemed to infuse me with a crystal clarity of perception, an ability to comprehend and understand aspects of life that usually were confusing or unclear. While out walking, I passed many older, retired people who had come to Bright for the autumn experience. I observed how happy, relaxed, and lively they appeared to be. There seemed to be magic in the place and in the experience that was unfolding.

As was my habit, after walking for an hour or so, I stopped at a wooden table by the beautiful river that runs through Bright and pondered the wonder of the place. I took out my notebook and began to write. I was considering what it was about Bright that contributed to my newfound clarity of vision and renewed energy. The town is nestled in a valley between mountains, and I thought that this could be a significant factor. Perhaps there were underground streams or significant ley lines that enhanced the energy? As I continued to speculate on paper with more ideas, ranging far and wide in plausibility, a continuous interruption was taking place. Under the influence of a gentle breeze, the tree beneath which I sat and several others nearby were dropping leaves all over the table. At regular intervals, there was a direct hit on my A4 notebook. I had to repeatedly sweep the leaves from my writing surface. I regarded them at this point as a mere annoyance.

Under this barrage of falling leaves, "Newton's apple" was bound to drop sooner or later. The idea flashed across my mind that perhaps some of the qualities I was experiencing in Bright were due to the essences or energy of these falling leaves. My first response was to reject this notion outright. The energies of flower essences I knew and loved. If falling leaves had a useful energy or essence about them, they would surely have been discovered, characterized, and promoted long ago. Other objections followed quickly from my scientifically trained intellect. Falling leaves are a spent force; their life and vitality lie in time past rather than time present. Surely they could have little if any nourishment left in them. Many are dehydrated and shriveled—hardly a promising starting point for essence work.

After the initial realization and the numerous objections raised by the rational mind, inner stillness returned to me. With the intellect suspended, my awareness tuned to a finer level of subtle energy as I sat at the table. This awareness had been cultivated by years of working with and sensing the energies of flower essences and homeopathic remedies. It seemed to me that, along with the physical bombardment of falling leaves, there was a fine golden light, imperceptible earlier, that streamed down from the trees above. I picked up a leaf and held it in my hand. A tingling sensation ran through my hand and up my arm. It was similar to the sensation I felt when I picked up a flower essence or homeopathic remedy bottle. My senses were detecting an energy or essence associated with the fallen leaf.

As I pondered this energy and began to wonder what type of energy a fallen leaf would have, the following words rose to my mind: *releasing the old, letting go of the past.* I considered the experience of the leaf as it fell from the tree. Leaving behind the safety and life it had known, the leaf completely separates from the tree and enters free fall. If a leaf were sufficiently conscious, that might be a very scary experience! Upon landing, the leaf gradually composts and is returned to the earth. Remembering the Doctrine of Signatures, this gave me a grasp of this essence type quickly. Falling leaf essences would aid in releasing and letting go and help one through the scary experience of "free fall," that fear that arises from change, when safety and security are left behind. Finally, this essence type would help integrate people more fully with the earth, because it is to the earth that the leaf falls. Every autumn thereafter, I felt drawn to Bright by an irresistible attraction. Each autumn the pilgrimage to Bright left me with fresh insight and awareness. Each autumn I collected more falling leaves, initially from Bright but then also from Melbourne and other places. Trudi Dempsey and later Jennie Richardson played a vital role not only in collecting but also in identifying leaves and in intuiting the action of some of the falling leaf essences.

Over the years, I have used these falling leaf essences successfully in my own practice. Other practitioners have used them as well. All have been delighted, perhaps even enchanted, with them. The overall response has been that not only do falling leaf essences work well in practice, but that also they are fundamentally different from other essence types currently available. In chapter 8, some of these practitioners will contribute their impressions and case histories of using the falling leaf essences.

Essences for the Four Seasons

The cycle of the four seasons is enacted in the daily lives of people everywhere. At times there is nothing much happening in a person's life, analogous to the dormancy of winter. There is the need to germinate some new endeavor or aspect of creativity. At other times a person is in a rapid growth phase in a particular area or in general. This is analogous to the spring season. At other times, there is a full bloom of creative expression, analogous to the summer. At other times, no further progress can be made in life until the person is able to release some aspect of the past. This is analogous to the autumn season.

Simply put, essence types should be matched seasonally with the current needs of the person. Seed essences are the basic essence type of winter; shoot essences are of spring; flower essences are of summer; and falling leaf essences are of autumn.

In deciding which type of seasonal essence to use, refer to diagram 3.1. For example, person A (Sarah) is a student who can't get going at all with a new course. She feels that she lacks connection to the material and is frustrated at her seeming inability to muster the willpower to overcome the problem. Of course, she could simply be struggling with laziness, yet an essence practitioner may decide the problem is genuine and select an appropriate essence. The practitioner refers to diagram 3.1 and asks, "Where on the seasonal cycle is Sarah?" Clearly Sarah is experiencing a state of dormancy; there's nothing happening in her life. This points the practitioner to the winter season, and Sarah (person A) is placed on diagram 3.1 in the winter season accordingly. Seed essences are the most promising essence type for Sarah. Once ingested, the seed essences may catalyze either a major change in attitude toward studying or, perhaps, a recognition that the course is inappropriate.

Person B (Peter) is an artist who gets started on a number of paintings

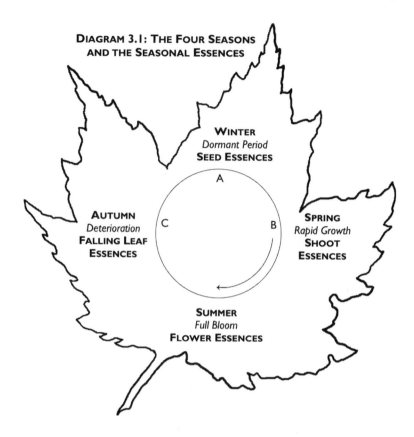

DIAGRAM 3.1: THE FOUR SEASONS
AND THE SEASONAL ESSENCES

WINTER
Dormant Period
SEED ESSENCES

A

AUTUMN
Deterioration
FALLING LEAF
ESSENCES

C

B

SPRING
Rapid Growth
SHOOT
ESSENCES

SUMMER
Full Bloom
FLOWER ESSENCES

but seems to lack the vital energy to bring these projects through to completion. An exhibition is scheduled, but at this rate the work will certainly not be completed in time. Peter is placed in the spring season on diagram 3.1. Clearly, the seed has germinated (the paintings are begun), but Peter lacks the vital expansion or creative energy that spring shoot essences are well able to provide. Later, flower essences may be suitable to bring the work to its completion, as Peter moves into summer on his creative cycle.

Person C (Bruce) has recently left a job but can't move on in life because he still feels so much anger toward his former employer and colleagues. Bruce is placed in the autumn season on diagram 3.1, because he needs to release the past emotionally. Falling leaf essences can greatly help Bruce let go of the intense emotions inspired by his past and move on.

It is important to clarify what *the four seasons* means here. On a calendar, the four seasons are each assigned a three months' duration. The seasons of the plant cycle usually, but not always, agree reasonably with the calendar seasons. Most flowering plants do so in summer, but some flower in autumn, spring, or even in winter. For our purposes, the four seasons follow the cycle of the individual plant. For example, a plant flowering in the calendar winter season is actually in its summer season. Thus, when we refer to flower essences being derived from the summer season, we mean the summer season of the plant cycle. Likewise, most deciduous trees shed their leaves in the calendar autumn season. But for those that shed their leaves in the calendar spring season, that calendar spring season is the autumn of the plant cycle.

Prescribing the Seasonal Essences

To claim that summer is a more important season than autumn or spring is clearly folly, because the seasons are interdependent. Likewise, it is folly to claim that flower essences are more important than falling leaf essences or seed essences. These essence types are interdependent, and each shows its best action when carefully selected according to the needs of the person. Table 3.1 shows the theoretical applicability of the four seasonal essence types to different types of problems or situations. As we will come to see later, in the case of not only flower essences but also falling leaf essences, there is a considerable body of practitioner experience to support this theory.

A Caution

Selecting essences based on the seasonal model is extremely simple. But what if an inappropriate essence type is selected? What if the person needs spring shoot essences but is prescribed seed essences instead? Generally speaking, if the inappropriate essence type is one season removed from the actual need, the person who takes it will still derive some benefit. Potentially more serious is the use of an essence type that is two seasons removed from the actual need. For example, a person may require falling leaf essences of autumn but is given shoot essences of spring. The essence may prove to be neither helpful nor harmful, but there may at times be an adverse action, because the type of energy is too far removed from the actual need.

TABLE 3.1: APPLICABILITY OF DIFFERENT SEASONAL ESSENCE TYPES IN DIFFERENT SITUATIONS

Situation	Applicability of Essence Type			
	Shoot Essences	Flower Essences	Falling Leaf Essences	Seed Essences
Anxiety	LOW	MEDIUM	HIGH	NIL
Depression	NIL	HIGH	MEDIUM	ADVERSE
Fatigue	NIL	LOW	MEDIUM	NIL
Hyperactivity	MEDIUM	HIGH	LOW	NIL
Leaving school or job	NIL	LOW	HIGH	NIL
Loneliness	NIL	LOW	MEDIUM	NIL
Need to detoxify physically	MEDIUM	NIL	HIGH	ADVERSE
Persistent anger	NIL	MEDIUM	HIGH	NIL
Physical injury (bruising)	NIL	NIL	LOW	NIL
Process of grieving	ADVERSE	LOW	HIGH	NIL
Relationship problems	NIL	MEDIUM	HIGH	NIL
Shock of accident and bereavement	NIL	HIGH	LOW	LOW
Sporting development (training)	LOW	NIL	LOW	MEDIUM
Starting a new course	HIGH	MEDIUM	NIL	HIGH
Starting a new relationship	HIGH	MEDIUM	NIL	HIGH

The effect of the essence is considered to be positive (low, medium, or high), neutral (nil), or negative (adverse). The effect is a general one for the type of situation described. One can no doubt point to particular examples that, considered in isolation, appear to contradict information in this table.

It is often argued that essences, being nontoxic, are completely safe and harmless to use. This notion of harmlessness is then used to support careless or unthinking use of essences on a "let's try it and see" basis. More true to reality is the recognition that essences are potentially strong energies that are capable of acting as potent disruptive forces in people's lives if used in inappropriate or unthinking ways. It was the American homeopath James Tyler Kent who lamented that he would rather be in a roomful of people slashing randomly with knives than in the presence of an ignorant prescriber of high-potency homeo-pathics. Homeopathy is certainly much more physical in its conse-quences than many other types of essences. But while the failures of flower essence therapy, for example, are not usually physical disasters, there is damage in the more subtle but no less real realms of emotion, mind, and spirit. This damage can result from using the inappropriate type of essence or essences that are too strong. Damage can even occur when essence therapy is continued for too long; inner change can be profoundly stressful, and most people need a significant break after a period of taking essences to facilitate inner change.

4 The Energetics of Falling Leaf Essences

WE'VE LEARNED THAT FALLING LEAF ESSENCES work well in assisting the process of releasing or letting go physically, mentally, emotionally, and spiritually. However, if one were to cut short the understanding of falling leaf essences at this point, a bigger picture is missed. Falling leaf essences bring about larger changes, as well, especially when a person has taken several different falling leaf essences over time. To understand these energetics that are general to the falling leaf essence category, we must first look at nature and the phenomenon of falling leaves in the autumn season.

The formation of a leaf by a tree is a common yet wonderful process. The tree draws its nourishment from the earth through its roots. These nutrients are assimilated by the plant and formed into leaves. Leaves are the site of photosynthesis, the process by which the tree derives from sunlight yet more energy.

However, in deciduous plants, as autumn approaches, shorter day length and colder temperatures render the leaves superfluous to the plant; it will remain partially dormant for the winter and will not need the energy of the sun. The green chlorophyll pigment breaks down, exposing the colors of the other pigments in the leaves. The leaves not only change color but also often become brittle or dry as the plant stops feeding them water and life-force energy. Eventually the leaves fall to the ground and are gradually composted back to earth from whence it came.

Ten Principles of Falling Leaf Energies

Clearly, an understanding of falling leaf essences needs to be based on the observation and interpretation of this natural cycle. Ten principles of falling leaf essence energetics can be drawn from this cycle, beyond the basic understanding of releasing and letting go developed in chapter 3.

✿ Principle One: Balance in Giving and Receiving

In the life cycle of the leaf, the leaf receives much nourishment and energy from the tree, which derives its nourishment from the earth. Using this nourishment, the leaf grows strong and then contributes to the well-being of the tree via photosynthesis. The falling leaf is the stage of its life cycle when it gives itself back to the earth. Only through this final stage of falling to the earth and being composted is the leaf's cycle of giving and receiving completed.

In the life cycle of human beings, through childhood and adolescence a young person receives much nourishment, particularly from immediate family but also significantly at school and from extended family and friends. Often parents and others make many sacrifices to ensure the best possible upbringing and opportunities for the developing child. Then a point of adulthood is reached where the person becomes independent and forms his or her own life. Now the person can either begin to give back to others and to society in various ways or pursue a selfish lifestyle, focused exclusively on personal goals. Falling leaf essences are a wake-up call for such self-centered people who are not giving back to the earth or society. Their action on this issue is subtle but persistent. For example, a person's conscience may become troubled because he or she has been neglecting a parent or elderly relative or because an intimate relationship runs much more based on his or her agenda and needs than that of his or her partner's. Sometimes a person will simply begin pondering the questions of what he or she can do to help the world in some small but meaningful way.

Falling leaf essences can also help give balance to those who give more than they receive. However, their primary strength is in cultivating giving, just as the falling leaf gives itself back to the earth.

🍂 Principle Two: Rebalancing the Ego

Falling leaf essences profoundly challenge and rebalance the ego. The human ego perceives itself to be separate from (and usually superior to) other human beings. Many philosophies and religions pronounce that all humans are really one in spirit and that separation is actually an illusion of the phenomenal world. Whether or not this is the case, the ego clings to a belief of separate existence and almost indestructible strength. Falling leaf essences challenge the notions of separate existence and perpetual strength. When the leaf falls back to the earth and is broken down, it loses its separate existence. Within a year or two it is usually integrated back into the soil. It simply no longer has a separate existence. It has become part of a greater whole. The leaf has also lost its vitality and strength. It has become so weak that it can no longer cling to the tree that has nourished it. The recognition and reality of fragility, aging, and death inherent in falling leaf essences is profoundly challenging to the ego. Through falling leaf essences, people come to an easier acceptance of aging and death, both metaphysical and physical.

🍂 Principle Three: Releasing Parental Bonds

A falling leaf has completely severed its connection to the parent tree. In entering free fall, it lets go of past attachment and differentiates itself from the tree. It now has a separate existence.

The separation of humans from their parents spans several decades. Though adults may no longer have a material need for their parents, at some level they may cling to the old parent-child bond. It can be scary to let go of apparent security, and that fear creates a continuing bond of dependence. The lingering dysfunctional bond might be emotional, mental, or even spiritual. The timely severing of outdated parent-child bonds usually brings improvement to the present-day relationship between parents and their adult children. The relationship is able to move to a different, more natural level, without the stress of past patterns that are no longer appropriate.

🍂 Principle Four: Bonding with the Earth

Because falling leaves return to the earth, their essences generate a unity with the earth. This may reflect in a person experiencing increased concern for the planet's welfare and for issues such as pollution and progressive extinction of flora and fauna. It may also reflect in a person's increased intimacy with and appreciation of nature. Falling leaf essences encourage in a person a longing to interact with nature and a greater willingness to allow time and energy for this to occur.

The essences' ability to connect people with the earth is a grounding ability. Falling leaf essences are therefore well suited for those people who tend to be airy-fairy, off in another world, and too much in their head. They tend to produce within people a very practical outlook, a way of problem solving that is based on practical realities and not so much on esoteric considerations.

🍂 Principle Five: Releasing Fear

Falling leaf essences are wonderful in assisting the release of a wide range of fears. They can help one to accept the sensation of free fall that accompanies fundamental change. In this capacity falling leaf essences are tremendously useful for all denizens of the world. As the pace of change we experience intensifies, we are all in free fall to varying extents, and none of us knows our destination. Falling leaf essences help eliminate the unease we feel for change, which is fundamentally fear.

The action of falling leaf essences is illustrated by holding a rubber ball in one hand. Squeeze this ball tightly, determined not to let it go. Imagine that something terrible could happen if you did! This act of squeezing the ball to ensure that it remains in your possession generates muscular tension, especially in the hand and forearm. If you continue squeezing the ball in this way for ten or fifteen minutes, you will probably find your posture changing unfavorably as compensation takes place in an effort to relieve tired muscles. Also, you will begin to feel tired. It takes a lot of energy to squeeze as determinedly as you are doing.

In this illustration, the muscular contraction represents fear in an emotional sense. Fear is a contracting emotion, and it generates muscular contraction in the physical body. If the fear of losing the rubber ball becomes more intense, the muscular contraction will become more intense also. Suppose now that you decide to release the ball. From your present state of muscular contraction in hand and forearm, note that it is impossible to release the rubber ball without relaxing your muscles. In fact, all you need to do is relax those muscle groups in hand and forearm and the rubber ball will be released and fall to the ground.

This simple illustration is profound in understanding the action of falling leaf essences and the role that fear plays. It is fear that causes us to hang on, and this fear causes contraction. Many people during or after falling leaf essence treatment report feeling a lot more relaxed in their body, as if the essences were some kind of muscle relaxant! Also, they report having much more energy. As we have seen, falling leaf essences are not regarded as strengthening or rebalancing essences. How I interpret the extra energy is that previously this energy was being used up in the process of hanging on grimly, as with the rubber ball in the above illustration. Now that energy is freed up and available! The rubber ball example also illustrates that fear is the pivotal emotion that causes us to hang on. It is in lessening and in mobilizing this fear into action that falling leaf essences excel. They are the catalyst that causes us to release the contraction and let go of the rubber ball.

🍂 Principle Six: Releasing Deep Trauma

Falling leaf essences can also assist people in releasing deep traumas that they may not even be aware of. Although a particular falling leaf essence might be prescribed to help a person let go of or release something on a more superficial level, if a person is ready, he or she will sometimes use this energy at a soul level to release something much deeper.

When the soul is ready for this release, all probably will be well. However, the practitioner of falling leaf essences needs to be aware that the essences have the potential to inspire deeper-than-intended release. The practitioner should also be aware that falling leaf essences are inappropriate for people who are addicted to emotional or psychological suffering. These people might subconsciously use the essence to dredge up past issues and emotions in an untimely and maximally dramatized fashion. Unless they have a sufficient level of self-awareness to acknowledge and cooperate in changing this pattern, such people should not use falling leaf essences.

🍂 Principle Seven: Understanding the Bigger Picture

Falling leaf essences afford one a detached perspective and enhanced understanding of processes of change and release in the world. That is, under the influence of a falling leaf essence, one at times gets a glimpse of "the bigger picture." One is brought to an awareness that a change one contemplates is much more than a personal decision and becomes aware of a certain larger responsibility inherent in a decision. If, for example, a person feels it is appropriate to move from one place to another or change jobs, he or she senses in this expanded state of consciousness that there is someone else intended to move in to his or her former place or post. The person realizes that if he or she does not make the intended move, this decision will hold back that other person.

One may prefer to believe that one's decisions to change or not to change are purely personal and do not have an impact on others. The expanded consciousness promoted through falling leaf essences demonstrates the fallacy of such insular thinking. With the power of choice comes responsibility. With the power of choice come implications for self as well as others. One can be a positive catalyst of change in the world or an obstacle, like a roadblock.

🍂 Principle Eight: Metaphysical Insight

Inherent in all falling leaf essences is the ability to give metaphysical insight into the problem being treated. For example, a person might be treated for persistent nausea with the appropriate falling leaf essence. He or she may not only improve physically but also come to the realization that the nausea is being caused by some aspect of life that is out of balance or requires attention. The first wave of action of the essence is to grant improvement or relief. The second wave is to grant understanding. Of course, these two aspects can occur simultaneously.

In giving understanding or insight, it seems that the action of falling leaf essences is to take the person into a more detached third-person observer position in relation to the self.

✤ Principle Nine: Spiritual Vision

A falling leaf essence encapsulates a kind of death experience. When a leaf is attached to the tree, one could consider it to be alive; when it is detached, in a sense it is dead, yet it continues to have an essence, one that is different from that of the attached leaf. In a sense, a falling leaf essence is "from the other side," the essence of something that has died. Therefore, it can confer an increased sensitivity to the realms of the dead, or the spirit world, an invisible realm of energy and experience of which most people are unaware. In particular, an increased sense of the angelic realm may emerge.

This increased spiritual perception does not become excessive, such that it might unduly distract a person from daily life, because falling leaf essences are simultaneously quite grounding. A person using falling leaf essences may have an increased perception and awareness of heaven, but his or her feet will be planted on the earth more firmly than ever.

✤ Principle Ten: Kundalini

Kundalini is a fire energy that moves up and down the spine. As it moves, sometimes with intensity, it clears energy blockages. This clearing process can produce a variety of psychological and physical symptoms. In many Eastern spiritual disciplines, kundalini is seen as a path to enlightenment. Kundalini is less understood in Western culture; it is often completely overlooked as an explanation for intense symptoms. Kundalini is essentially associated with the spine, and nerves from the spine radiate to the entire body. Therefore, symptoms generated by kundalini might be felt in any part of the body, and might mimic those of many different illnesses. It simply doesn't fit the Western way of thinking about symptoms and causation.

It is generally recognized that certain types of meditation and yoga practices stimulate kundalini. Kundalini can also be awakened by falling leaf essences, most commonly when two or three are prescribed in sequence. Generally the awakening of kundalini is not a problem—unless it has already been awakened. This may be the case when a person is taking flower essences, which also have, to a lesser extent, a tendency to awaken kundalini. If the person or practitioner believes that kundalini has been awakened, it is usually better to avoid falling leaf essences until the kundalini settles. A very uncomfortable intensity can be generated by superimposing the action of falling leaf essences on top of an already active kundalini.

Falling leaf essences' tendency to awaken kundalini may relate to their earth connection. One way of looking at kundalini esoterically is that it represents a flow of energy from earth to heaven and back again. The flow begins at the base chakra (earth), flows to the crown chakra (heaven), and then flows back down again. A falling leaf's energy is clearly moving downward from the crown of the tree to the earth, under the influence of gravity. Yet the falling leaf aspires to raise its energy back to reconnect to the tree. Thus, the energy of the falling leaf essence is upward from the earth back toward the crown. This desire of the leaf to reattach to the tree generates an upward-flowing energy stream that stimulates kundalini in the body.

The Love Factor

The ten principles outlined above describe the many varied ways in which falling leaf essences clear the body of blockages and unresolved issues. It's all this clearing, I believe, that leads to a striking change: People develop an increased capacity to give and receive love. A heart filled with fear, anger, and greed cannot simultaneously be filled with love. But as falling leaf essences empty out these feelings, the capacity to love increases.

Because falling leaf essences detoxify the system not just physically but mentally and emotionally as well, they act as powerful preventives of disease. Yet their action is far greater than this and extends to social levels of interaction. When we become emotionally and mentally toxic, through accumulation of emotional intensity around issues, beliefs, and events that we cannot or will not release and let go of, we experience a distancing from people around us. These people learn that either they need to avoid certain subjects altogether when they are interacting with us, lest they experience our mental and emotional toxicity verbally or energetically, or they brace themselves for a verbal fight. In either case, the free flow of the interaction is halted. Distance is generated. Intimacy or communion is lost, and the ability to give or receive love is at least temporarily suspended.

It cannot be overstated that the outcome of a falling leaf essence prescription is unpredictable. It is always difficult to isolate the cause and effect of change in people's lives. Sometimes the prescription seems to alter only the area in which help was sought. In other cases, it seems as if the falling leaf essence was like placing a stick in a river, driving it into the sand at just the right point. This small stick in the river alters the whole flow pattern of the river, such that it begins to take an entirely new course downstream.

How Do Falling Leaf Essences Work?

It is interesting to speculate as to how falling leaf essences actually work. A great deal of basic research is needed to elucidate the mode of action of an essence on the human organism. Because there is currently a complete absence of evidence as to the biochemical action of falling leaf essences, one has complete freedom to speculate!

The Molecular Hypothesis

During the process of preparing falling leaf essences, the leaves exude certain compounds, including pigments, into the essence. The notion that these compounds are what enable falling leaf essences to exert their influence could be called the molecular hypothesis. However, it is difficult to believe that the action of falling leaf essences could be explained solely by the molecular hypothesis. The essence stock is greatly diluted; just a few drops are used in preparing 25 and 50 ml bottles of essence for ingestion.

✿ The Energetic Signature Hypothesis

The leaves could also release subtle energy, a kind of energetic imprint or remnant similar to that which is postulated to occur in homeopathy. In homeopathy, as explained in chapter 1, some kind of subtle energy *must* be involved, because preparations that can be shown using Avogadro's number to have no molecules at all are still biologically active with patients. This notion that falling leaf essences operate on a level of subtle energy could be called the energetic signature hypothesis. There are several lines of logic that go beyond the scope of this section that point to the energetic signature hypothesis as being highly credible. The natural question arising from this discussion is what the nature of this subtle energy is and how it affects the living cell. Possibly the twenty-first century will see the extension of science into realms of subtle energy that were previously the exclusive domain of mystics and hypersensitive individuals.

✿ Biochemical Hypotheses

As I come from a biochemical background, I have over time developed hypotheses as to how falling leaf essences influence the living cell. Perhaps they act primarily as catalysts for certain reactions within the cell. (Catalysts are substances that speed up a chemical reaction but do not alter its outcome.) These hypotheses are:

1. Falling leaf essences stimulate RNA replication in the cell.
2. They act potently at the level of the ribosome to promote protein synthesis.
3. They stimulate the metabolic rate by operating on the Krebs cycle.
4. They promote the expulsion of toxic materials and waste products from the cytoplasm.
5. They strengthen the cell membrane by acting on the lipid layers.

✿ The "Essence Reserve"

Another hypothesis, to date devoid of supporting evidence but still a fruitful idea for further investigation, concerns the human body's ability to store essences. In the physical realm the human body converts excess carbohydrates and fats into storable fat. These fat reserves can then be drawn upon later, in times when there is less food available or physical demands are greater. (This has become a problem in the modern world, where food is always plentifully available and the fat reserves are continually being laid down!) On the energetic level, it may be that the body uses subtle energies that are present in the environment but stores them—in the spinal fluid or the pancreas, perhaps—when they are available at levels in excess of need. Later, when the system experiences extreme stress—for example, an accident, an illness, or surgery—this reservoir is called upon. This hypothesis may partly explain why people who take essences frequently appear to have more ability to "bounce back" from illness or accident.

⚘ Essences and the Endocrine System

The notion that falling leaf essences assist in releasing and letting go of the old suggests that they have an affinity for the body's endocrine system. This is because the body clocks of the endocrine system govern processes of acquisition and release of biological materials and their relative rates. Through its hormone-producing glands, the endocrine system governs the body's internal clocks. As the human body experiences the different seasons of the year, internal physical adjustments take place, triggered by the changing length of the light period, the changing temperature, and the changing availability of food. Falling leaf essences could be a kind of cue for the body to adjust the balance of the body clocks that keep track of the seasons. That is, whenever a falling leaf essence is ingested, the system goes through a review of the appropriateness of the settings of the different body clocks.

Falling leaf essences are helpful for adjusting endocrine problems, which frequently arise when the system is having difficulty coping with the pace and extent of change—"I can't keep up!" Big life changes, such as moving overseas, moving to a new house, beginning or ending a relationship, buying or selling property, and often a complex of these and other stresses, call for falling leaf essences to help the endocrine system cope. Of course, the endocrine system governs the stress response, the "fight or flight" reaction, and can therefore suffer burnout after prolonged stress.

✿ The Rest Cycle

In some cases, falling leaf essences cause people to feel quite tired. People who go, go, go and do not allow adequate time for rest, relaxation, and rebalancing may find themselves low in energy for quite a while after taking these essences. Falling leaf essences seem to bring to the surface long-suppressed tiredness and exhaustion. They seem to carry within them the understanding that it is appropriate to have both periods of high energy and periods of relative rest and relaxation. Autumn is the season in which nature is beginning to slow down to prepare for winter. Falling leaf essences, the essences of autumn, in turn encourage people who are overwrought and overstressed to slow down.

✿ The Interpersonal Connection

It has been established through long experience that homeopathics and flower essences are basically personal essences. That is, these essences produce change on a strictly personal level. Obviously, if a person changes, that person's relationships with other people also change, to some extent, so as a secondary result homeopathics and flower essences may have interpersonal effects. Falling leaf essences appear to be essentially different in that their action often seems to extend to a group of about four to twenty people. How can this be, if only one person is ingesting the essence?

We have invisible, energetic connections to those people who are close to us. Some are family members, while others are friends. Perhaps some kinds of essences are able to radiate along these lines of interconnection. Another way of expressing this possibility is that the energy of letting go and releasing could be infectious! It has certainly been my frequent experience to hear a client tell me that, after beginning a program of falling leaf essences, his or her whole family, group of friends, or intimate relationship is going through profound transformation. Clearly, not only the person taking the essence but others as well are releasing and changing. Pendulum dowsing also suggests that falling leaf essences have the ability to act at a group level. This needs to be borne in mind by the practitioner.

🍂 The Danger of Projection

At times, a consequence of ingesting falling leaf essences is that some intensity arises from the past. It may be a difficult issue that has raised its head, it could be a troublesome emotion, or it could be a lingering trauma. It could even be that the falling leaf essences tapped in to some joy or ecstasy from the past that is quite uncomfortable in its intensity! There comes a critical moment in which either we own and take responsibility for that which has come forth or we seek to find someone or something outside ourselves to blame or hold responsible. We could argue that if the difficult emotion is from childhood, then it is our parents' fault. Or if the intensity takes us by surprise, it could be the therapist's fault for giving us an essence that was "far too strong." Or if the dissatisfaction arises due to our career, then it could be the boss's fault, and even political figures such as local government or national leaders could cop the blame.

However, we must all take responsibility for our own lives. The almost universal tendency to hold someone else responsible for our own intensities is both childish and ultimately futile. Once we transfer responsibility from ourselves to someone else, once we hold someone else responsible and act as judge and jury together over him or her, then we have denied ourselves the potential benefit of the releasing and letting-go process. In fact, the process of releasing and letting go stops in the very instant we transfer responsibility elsewhere. Rather than letting go, we then hold on to the emotion or the issue, fiercely. We need to hold on in order to continue to pronounce the accused guilty with the full intensity of our righteous indignation. This pattern of holding other people, groups, and causes responsible for our own problems, past or present, is so universal that it also occurs on a local and national level in the media, where unfortunate individuals and groups are often set up as the scapegoats for the sufferings of humanity at large. By contrast, an individual who owns and takes responsibility for his or her own beliefs, attitudes, and emotions presents a pleasing and refreshing picture.

5 A Compendium of Falling Leaf Essences

THE PROCESS OF DEDUCING THE ACTION and role of a falling leaf essence occurs initially on an intuitive level. Even as one finds a suitable tree, collects the falling leaves, and prepares the essence, there may already be a developing sense of the nature and role of the resulting essence. At other times one may sit down in a quiet and relaxed setting, pen and paper ready, to intuitively access information.

There is nothing objectionable about the intuitive model, so long as the intuitive information is held with a healthy skepticism. Both the essences and the information about them must always be "proved," or verified in practice, not only by the essence preparer but also by other practitioners. Repeated feedback from many clients who have taken this essence over time builds up a picture of the scope, reliability, and usefulness of the essence. Indeed, this is how Edward Bach began with his flower essences.

When describing falling leaf essences to people, the most commonly asked question is how the information about the action of each essence comes into being. The following simple model assists understanding.

Diagram 5.1 shows a sphere that represents different states of consciousness. The outside surface of the sphere could be regarded as a portal or membrane that one must cross to reach the altered levels of consciousness within. Point X outside the sphere represents normal everyday waking consciousness. In this state of consciousness, one is

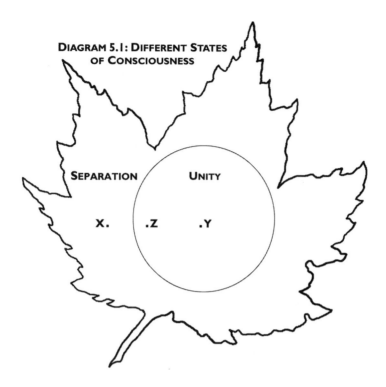

DIAGRAM 5.1: DIFFERENT STATES
OF CONSCIOUSNESS

SEPARATION   UNITY

X.   .Z   .Y

aware of seemingly separate objects and events in the perceptual or visible world. This is a consciousness in which logic, calculation, and reason may predominate. Point Y at the center of the sphere represents a consciousness wherein there exists no separation. Everything is perceived as an aspect of one. At point Y there is awareness but no words; understanding is felt and perhaps seen but not spoken. There is immediate and seemingly effortless access to information or understanding that is unavailable in the normal state of everyday consciousness represented by point X. The sense of interconnectedness and unity of all things at point Y is so strong that the adjustment to the normal separated state of consciousness represented by point X is profound and not always quickly or easily accomplished.

There is nothing novel about the ideas represented in diagram 5.1. They have been discussed and experienced for thousands of years, especially in the East, but also in some branches of Christianity. Point Y is sometimes referred to as the cosmic or universal consciousness. In esoteric Christianity, it might be referred to as the divine or Christ consciousness. Historical examples of individuals who have reached point Y in a "spiritual experience" abound. Sometimes they are unable to speak for many days (recall that there are no words at point Y), and they often gain unique information or revelation out of the experience. An example might be the experience of the apostle Paul on the Damascus Road.

Accessing point Y is not an experience for the uninitiated. It is profoundly stressful to move suddenly from point X to point Y when one has not done it before. The huge change of consciousness is like the sudden decompression of a deep-sea diver or a parachute jumper from high above the ground. The result can be profound and lasting disorientation, inability to communicate, and, in extreme cases, lasting psychological or psychiatric disorders. Individuals who have done years of consistent meditation, yoga, prayer, pendulum dowsing, or another suitable practice are able reach this point Y consistently and without effort. However, only a minority of people, even after prolonged training, can reach point Y and return with a crystal clarity and the extreme accuracy required for many scientific inventive purposes.

In terms of falling leaf essences, point X—normal consciousness—is the state in which one would collect the leaves and make the essence. Then by moving to point Y, one could come to know at a deep and assured place within oneself what this essence was useful for. However, at point Y one finds understanding but no words. How, then, can one communicate the understanding to other people? There is a third point, Z, that lies within the sphere but more toward the periphery. At this point, there is a degree of separation from the unity of Y. At this point, one is able to use words—the voice of the separated consciousness—while still in tune with Y, the point of unity in which understanding of the essence is made clear.

Three understandings are essential to complete this picture. The first is that over time, with repeated practice at changing the level of consciousness from point X to point Y and to Z, there comes the ability to embrace these different levels of consciousness simultaneously. That is, one can be aware of the separate objects and ideas of the visible world, aware of the understanding of this that goes beyond words, and also aware of how to express it. The second point is that whatever information or understanding emerges from this process of changing consciousness must be turned over to the skeptical, rational mind and tested in whatever ways are possible. Intuited information should never be accepted as if it were a divine decree! The third understanding is that accessing information of significance to the progress of humanity can be a perilous undertaking. The energetics involved in accessing significant inventions are volatile. The energetic disturbances generated can easily explode or implode into the life of the inventor, at the time of accessing or subsequently. Remember that at point X, one is dealing with personal energy. At point Y, one is dealing with universal or cosmic energy. The eruption of cosmic energy into the personal level can be extreme. To some extent, this can be minimized through the experience of the inventor.

How to Use the Listings in This Chapter

The falling leaf essences listed below are available from my company, Advanced Alchemy Pty. Ltd. And the numbering system is my own. These essences have been extensively tested and approved in the experience of many different practitioners. In describing these essences, one must bear in mind the many and various means by which practitioners select essences for their clients. These can be listed as follows:

1. The written description of the action of the essence, compared with the stated or perceived need of the client
2. Kinesiology (muscle testing)
3. Pendulum dowsing
4. Essence cards, which are shuffled and then randomly selected by the practitioner or client
5. The attraction a client feels toward photographs of trees, flowers, or other relevant plant parts from which the essence was created
6. Electronic testing (Mora, Thera, or Vega machines)

I believe strongly in the value of having more than one and, preferably, several different ways of arriving at an essence prescription. The beauty of having several approaches is that they sometimes give somewhat different results. That is excellent, because it really gets you thinking!

The first twenty-five essences described below are a representative selection of commonly applicable falling leaf essences, and they form a suitable "mini-kit." The mini-kit is an ideal introduction to falling leaf essences. These are the essences that encapsulate what falling leaf essences are all about. They represent the most commonly used falling leaf essences, and are selected to cover the diversity of physical, emotional, and mental problems that these essences are capable of treating. Although some people prefer to purchase the entire 160 essences in the falling leaf essence range, generally it is better to purchase twenty-five or fifty essences. One can then "get to know" these essences well and further essences can then be ordered individually as required. The first fifty represent the standard falling leaf essence kit. Falling leaf essences 51 through 160 have been added over the years as practitioners have requested more essences for particular purposes.

Please note that every reasonable step has been taken to ensure that the common and botanical names of the trees listed below are correct. This list has been painstakingly researched by a qualified horticulturist, but there is always a possible uncertainty about classification of trees, and the naming of some cultivars or varieties is controversial.

All the falling leaf essences are assigned a number; FLE 1, for example, is shorthand for falling leaf essence Claret Ash. All falling leaf essences are accompanied by the naming of an ailment or condition, such as "influenza" for FLE 1, "tonic" for FLE 2, "bereavement" for FLE 3, "osteoarthritis" for FLE 9, and "after stroke" for FLE 59. These titles note the condition or situation that each particular falling leaf essence is best suited for. If the falling leaf essence is best suited for a particular condition, such as influenza, osteoarthritis, or stroke, it may assist recovery or encourage improvement. What is meant by these titles is that the relevant falling leaf essence may assist recovery or encourage improvement in the corresponding condition. We are *not* claiming that FLE 1 is a cure for influenza, or that FLE 9 is a cure for osteoarthritis, or that FLE 59 will cure the aftereffects of stroke. Sometimes falling leaf essences will cure a condition, sometimes they will bring a large or modest improvement, and occasionally they won't work. That's just reality.

For a quick look through the actions of the essences, turn to table 5.1 (at the end of this chapter), which lists the core action for the 160 essences. Those interested in particular trees will find tables 5.2 (alphabetical listing by common name) and 5.3 (alphabetical listing by botanical name) useful references. An index of emotions and the falling leaf essences suited for assisting with them can be found in table 5.4, and the same treatment of physical complaints is given in table 5.5.

Those essences that act mostly on a physical level are denoted by a "P" next to their heading. Those that act mostly on a psychological (mental and emotional) level are denoted by an "M," and those that act mostly on a spiritual level are denoted by an "S." If there is no designation, then the essence does not fit neatly into just one of these categories.

Please note that in the vast majority of cases (in excess of 90 percent), the same essence prepared from the same tree in different locations shows virtually the same characteristics and activity. Very occasionally, however, one finds that a tree in a particular location produces an essence that is significantly different from the essence produced from similar specimens of the same tree elsewhere. Presumably some unique aspect or aspects of the environment are responsible. In this case the tree is indicated in the following list by a location in brackets. One case is afforded by Liquidamber, which essence has its usual action when prepared from the location Donvale (FLE 10 below), but an unusual and interesting action when prepared from a different location, Kallista (FLE 151). Another case is afforded by Cut-leaf Norway Maple, which has its standard action when prepared from the location Emerald (FLE 118), but the essence is distinctly different when prepared from the location Sherbrooke (FLE 61).

FLE 1   Claret Ash ♦ *Fraxinus angustifolia* 'Raywood'
Influenza ♦ P

This essence is used primarily for treating influenza. Claret Ash promotes the release of the virus via urine, bowel movement, and sweating. It eases the aches and pains that often accompany influenza and reduces the risk of secondary infections. When the infection has run its course, the essence helps the person feel quite well, rather than depleted or run down. A person should continue taking the essence for one week after the symptoms of viral infection are gone.

This essence also promotes a general detoxification of the system. The release of significant toxins or stored wastes occurs when an adult is given the essence at a dosage of 7 drops four to six times daily. When using the essence in this manner, symptoms similar to cold or influenza may ensue; this is a sign that the system is purging itself of waste products. In this case, the essence should be continued until all such symptoms cease.

FLE 2   Linden ♦ *Tilia* x *europea*
Tonic ♦ P

This essence is a great pick-me-up after a period of stress or after illness. It can also be taken on a continual basis to help in coping with ongoing stress. It strengthens and tones the adrenal glands, kidneys, nervous system, heart, and lungs.

FLE 3   Dove Tree ♦ *Davidia involucrata*
Bereavement

This is the classic falling leaf essence to give to a person who has recently lost a loved one. In the initial stage of shock, Bach's Rescue Remedy is unsurpassed. However, within two to four days, it is generally better to move on to Dove Tree falling leaf essence. This essence facilitates movement through the different emotional stages of grieving, ensuring that the person does not become stuck at any particular point.

FLE 4   Turkey Oak ♦ *Quercus cerris*
Endocrine System ♦ P

This essence works on all the major glands of the endocrine system, unblocking and balancing them. Therefore, it is of assistance in a great diversity of physical problems that stem from imbalances in the endocrine and hormonal systems of the body.

FLE 5   Weeping Willow ♦ *Salix babylonica*
Kidneys ♦ P

This essence works primarily on the kidneys, bladder, and urinary tract. Its action on the kidneys is to release toxins and rebalance. It offers assistance in the treatment of urinary tract infections, kidney problems, fluid retention due to kidney imbalance, cystitis, urine retention, and poor urinary flow (when not due to other physical problems such as enlarged prostate).

FLE 6   English Hawthorn ♦ *Crataegus laevigata*
Stomach and Pancreas ♦ P

English Hawthorn is useful for balancing hydrochloric acid production in the stomach, and it assists in repairing and maintaining the stomach lining. It also acts homeostatically on both digestive enzyme and insulin production by the pancreas. Accordingly, this essence should be considered in cases of chronic bad breath, chronic indigestion, Crohn's disease, dyspepsia, flatulence, and abdominal muscle cramps.

FLE 7   Cherry Plum ♦ *Prunus cerasifera*
Emotional Well-being

This essence helps address surface emotional issues and promotes a sense of emotional well-being. It is an outstanding feel-good essence. It is a good place to start when one wants to explore deeper emotional issues. It is also an essence to consider in the case of psychosomatic illness, for which it can benefit the physical symptoms.

FLE 8   Pin Oak ♦ *Quercus palustris*
Fatigue ♦ M

Pin Oak essence addresses fatigue due to mental stress and exhaustion. It slows down excessive irrelevant thought patterns and relaxes the mind. Pin Oak essence has a regenerative effect on nervous system tissue.

FLE 9   White Ash ♦ *Fraxinus americana*
Osteoarthritis ♦ P

Osteoarthritis is extremely common in older people. White Ash helps by increasing energy supply to joints, improving the release of waste products, and, to an extent, regenerating healthier joint tissue. The essence is therefore useful in osteoarthritis treatment and can be continued on a long-term basis if necessary.

FLE 10   Liquidamber (Donvale) ♦ *Liquidambar styraciflua*
Inflammation ♦ P

This essence counteracts inflammation in different parts of the body, so is to be seriously considered in inflammatory states, such as those of arthritis, chronic cough, enteritis, foot and leg ulcers, gastroenteritis, hepatitis, laryngitis, pleurisy, pneumonia, skin conditions, and tennis elbow.

FLE 11   English Elm ♦ *Ulmus procera*
Female Reproductive System ♦ P

The primary action of this essence is in assisting symptoms associated with menopause, including hot flashes, night sweats, dry hair or skin, and depression. The essence is also useful in balancing menstruation. It has a beneficial action with premenstrual tension and irregular or unduly heavy periods.

English Elm exerts its action on the hormonal systems of the body, including the pituitary, hypothalamus, ovary, and parathyroid glands.

FLE 12   Willow Pattern Tree (Golden Rain Tree) ♦ *Koelreuteria paniculata*
Nervous Insomnia ♦ M

Taken on an hourly basis, Willow Pattern Tree will lessen excessive mental activity that might otherwise prevent or detract from a good night's sleep. The essence promotes drowsiness and sleep.

FLE 13   Pink Horse Chestnut ♦ *Aesculus* x *carnea*
Fluid Retention ♦ P

This essence works on the renal system, pancreas, pituitary, hypothalamus, and lymphatic system to help in cases of fluid retention.

FLE 14   Apricot ♦ *Prunus armeniaca*
Release Anger ♦ M

This apricot essence operates at the subconscious mental level, allowing the release of held anger. This emotional release not only may benefit the person mentally and emotionally, but also may alleviate a physical condition to the extent that suppressed anger affected it.

FLE 15   Domestic Fig ♦ *Ficus carica* 'White Adriatic'
Release Guilt ♦ M

Domestic Fig operates to release mental control over guilt. Guilt is often related to low self-esteem and the notion of not being good enough. Since guilt is frequently associated with the idea of punishment, people who feel guilty will often punish themselves! The release of guilt stimulated by the essence may benefit the person mentally, emotionally, and/or physically.

FLE 16   Oriental Plane ♦ *Platanus orientalis*
Release Fear of Change ♦ M

This essence promotes the release of fear of change. This fear is practically universal, as it is inspired by the various unknowns that change brings and the apparent loss of safety and security associated with it. Yet the one certainty in life is change; we are unable to avoid it. This essence helps us enter the experience of the autumn leaf's free fall with trust and hope.

FLE 17   Weeping Katsura Tree ♦
Cercidiphyllum japonicum f. *pendulum*
Release Fear of Love ♦ S

The fear of love is one of the primary human fears. How can people fear that which they seem to want most in life? Fear of unconditional love can be based in part on low self-esteem and the fear of real intimacy. Weeping Katsura Tree releases and soothes this fear so that love can be faced with courage.

FLE 18   Copper Beech ♦ *Fagus sylvatica* 'Purpurea'
Release Hatred ♦ M

Hatred is, of course, a potently destructive force, not only in the life of a person who is hated, but also in the life of the one who chooses to hate. Hatred is a cancer of the human spirit. It unleashes potent psychic forces and wastes precious energetic resources. Life is truly too short to be wasted on negative emotions. Copper Beech is a precious gift to us and assists those who choose to release hatred.

FLE 19   Yellow Flowering Currant (Golden Currant) ♦
Ribes odoratum
Self-Esteem ♦ S

This is the first falling leaf essence to think of in cases of disablingly low self-esteem. It releases the core disbelief in self reflected in the statement "I can't." "I can't" can be the core problem in not moving forward in life, in not attempting that which is appropriate, or in not persevering with that which is started. The action of this essence, with support and encouragement, can result in a new momentum and direction in life.

FLE 20   Winter Hazel ♦ *Corylopsis sinensis* var. *calvescens*
Release Programmed Living ♦ S

Winter Hazel releases the need to live in a way that satisfies the expectations of parents, family, and society. Hence, it is particularly useful for impressionable people who lack the resolve to go against the judgment of those around them when they perceive a clear inner voice to follow another path. The essence imparts the strength to be oneself and to follow a truly suitable path in life, regardless of external pressures.

FLE 21   Lombardy Poplar ♦ *Populus nigra* var. *italica*
Substance Addiction ♦ S

This essence applies to cases of major substance addiction. It helps release the deep thought patterns and psychological needs underlying substance addiction. It assists with addictions to cigarettes, heroin, marijuana, and other medical and street drugs. The essence can be given before, during, and after substance withdrawal for up to three months in total. A typical dosage is 5 drops four times daily.

FLE 22   Glory Vine ♦ *Vitis coignetiae*
Release Mental Control ♦ M

Glory Vine releases the tendency of the mind to seek to direct and control life experience. In doing so, it enables one to live from the level of spirit rather than the level of mind. This generates a more natural flow of life with the exertion of much less energy. The mind, though still useful, can rest in the assurance that all is well. The essence is useful for those who are on a spiritual path but have active, intelligent minds that pose as many problems for their owners as they solve.

FLE 23   Black Pussy Willow ♦ *Salix* x *reichardtii* 'Nigra'
Specific Low Self-Esteem ♦ S

This essence releases the notion that one does not have the required ability to succeed in a particular area of life. Such a notion is usually based not on reality, but rather on some past criticism or insecurity. Black Pussy Willow differs from Yellow Flowering Currant (FLE 19) in that that the latter is for a generalized state of low self-esteem, whereas this essence is for low self-esteem only in a particular area of life.

FLE 24   Sawtooth Oak (Bristle-tipped Oak) ♦
Quercus acutissima
"Stiff Upper Lip" ♦ M

This essence is for those who have been programmed from childhood to have to be emotionally "held in" or suppressed. Sawtooth Oak releases a switch at the subconscious level to allow a broad spectrum of emotions to be felt and expressed. Use continually for three to six months in stubborn cases.

FLE 25   Elderberry ♦ *Sambuccus nigra*
Sexuality ♦ S

Elderberry catalyzes the release of restrictions and difficulties about sexuality. The essence allows the expression of love in a natural way without guilt and with full feeling.

FLE 26   Tulip Tree ♦ *Liriodendron tulipifera*
Heart ♦ P

Tulip Tree essence strengthens and balances the action of the heart. It may be of some use in treating atherosclerosis in its earlier stages, and it is beneficial in cases of angina. It is also useful in the prevention of heart disease and after heart surgery.

FLE 27   Persian Witch Hazel (Persian Ironwood) ♦
Parrotia persica
Release Children ♦ M

This essence assists in balancing emotions as they relate to emotional strangleholds on children. It can be helpful in situations where a child is being given up for adoption. It is also helpful in situations where parents have difficulty in allowing their adult children to journey on their own path in life.

FLE 28   Rowan ♦ *Sorbus aucuparia*
After Surgery ♦ P

This essence helps restore energy and repair damage after surgery. It assists in tissue repair and shortens the recovery period after general anesthetia.

FLE 29   Yeddo Cherry ♦ *Prunus yedoensis*
Mental Flexibility ♦ M

This essence assists particularly the not-so-young who have outdated and inflexible attitudes and beliefs. The essence releases rigid thought-forms and enables the person to entertain different ideas and to see another's point of view.

FLE 30   White Mulberry ♦ *Morus alba*
Muscular Weakness ♦ P

White Mulberry will help send energy to areas affected by muscle weakness, releasing toxins and reestablishing nutrient flow to the damaged tissue, which will help in the regeneration of tissue. This essence may assist in cases of hernia, prolapse of the uterus, and in muscular dystrophy.

FLE 31   Silver Birch ♦ *Betula pendula*
Release Struggle ♦ S

This is a wonderful essence for those who truly believe that life wasn't meant to be easy. Wherever there exists an addiction to a pattern of struggle in life, with an accompanying belief in scarcity and difficulty, this essence is called for. It releases these preconceived notions of difficulty and unblocks emotional barriers to abundance.

FLE 32   Silver Maple ✦ *Acer saccharinum*
Breasts ✦ P

A powerful lymphatic cleanser with an emphasis on breast tissue, silver maple is useful in the treatment of breast lumps, fluid retention, and hormonal imbalance.

FLE 33   Japanese Dogwood ✦ *Cornus kousa*
Gout ✦ P

This essence works by balancing uric acid production in proportion to the production of urine, thereby reducing the risk of excess uric acid forming into crystals. The essence will also address mental and emotional problems such as loss of interest in life, brooding, the "everything is too hard" feeling, "black cloud" syndrome, and the "what have I done to deserve this" feeling.

FLE 34   Plane Tree ✦ *Platanus racemosa*
Indigestion ✦ P

This essence will cause the pancreas to produce more digestive enzymes and balance the acid/alkaline nature of food in the stomach. It also has an action on the stomach, toning and balancing acidity.

FLE 35   Thornless Scarlet Honey Locust ✦
Gleditsia triacanthos 'Ruby Lace'
Release Disappointment ✦ M

Disappointment is the common emotional reaction when one's plans and hopes do not come to fruition. Because disappointment is not pleasant to experience, it is frequently obstructed or suppressed. In releasing disappointment, this essence helps one hope and have vision and trust in life once more.

FLE 36   Japanese White Birch ♦
Betula platyphylla var. *japonica*
Release Envy ♦ M

This essence applies to envy of another's gifts or abilities. Envy of another can be productive if that energy is channeled into expressing one's own potential and gifts in life. This emotion is negative when one sits back and stares enviously at another who is putting in the required effort and discipline to reap creative rewards. In that sense, suppressed envy is an "armchair" emotion that needs to be moved and expressed within one's own creative realm.

FLE 37   Thornless Golden Honey Locust ♦
Gleditsia triacanthos 'Sunburst'
Release Jealousy ♦ M

This essence particularly applies to jealousy of other people's material possessions or wealth. It releases an undue materialism and the mistaken notion that material wealth is a reflection of a person's innate value. In so doing, it generates an appreciation of the material things that one does have.

FLE 38   Red Crepe Myrtle ♦ *Lagerstroemia indica* 'Rubra'
Release Possessiveness ♦ M

It is a misconception to believe that we can ever possess or control another human being. Red Crepe Myrtle releases the emotions that have built up through this misconception of possessiveness and the emotional need to control others.

FLE 39   Aspen ♦ *Populus tremula*
Release Loneliness

Feelings of loneliness are very common. Aspen deals with intense feelings of loneliness that are disabling in some aspect of life. It enables one to face the world alone and without fear. In that sense, it confers full maturity and independence.

FLE 40   Chinese Trumpet Vine ✦ *Campsis grandiflora*
Release Fear of the Unknown ✦ M

Change takes us into unknown places, both within ourselves and externally in the world. It is a natural and universal human fear. Fear of the unknown is a real problem when it becomes disabling and actually obstructs a beneficial change from occurring. Fear of the unknown is exemplified by the free fall of the autumn leaf. Leaving the security of attachment to the tree, the leaf enters the terror of free fall, not knowing that Mother Earth awaits it. Chinese Trumpet Vine will not eliminate this fear, but it will reduce it to manageable proportions and transform it from an immobilizing to a mobilizing force.

FLE 41   Crepe Myrtle ✦ *Lagerstroemia indica*
Release Uncertainty

Feelings of uncertainty can at times prevent us from moving forward or from making a decision when one is clearly required. Crepe Myrtle resolves feelings of uncertainty stemming from the past, which enables a clear view of the issues and an unimpeded decision-making process.

FLE 42   Red Maple (Canadian Maple) ✦ *Acer rubrum*
Release Fear of Lack of Love ✦ M

This essence releases a belief that there is not enough love in the world and that love is in short supply. This can be a deep-rooted fear carried with us from childhood, when we feared that mother or father would desert us. This fear of there not being enough love can create repetitive addictive patterns of destructive relationships. It can also generate dysfunctional friendships that arise out of desperate emotional need rather than choice.

FLE 43   Chinese Elm ♦ *Ulmus parvifolia*
Release Inappropriate Individualism ♦ S
Releases the belief that "I, me, and mine" is the ultimate reality in life and in business. In releasing self-centered notions, Chinese Elm will enable a person to be a better team player, with the ability to empathize with others. In moving a person toward a solid notion of "we" instead of "I," it opens up thought and feeling for the group, the family, the society, and the world as a whole.

FLE 44   Weeping Elm ♦ *Ulmus glabra* 'Pendula'
Release Emotional Turmoil
Weeping Elm helps release a pattern of having periods of emotional turmoil or unpleasant emotions. Such a pattern may be held in the subconscious mind decades after its origin in a difficult childhood. This essence enables prolonged periods of emotional calm and enjoyment of life.

FLE 45   Port Wine Magnolia ♦ *Michelia figo*
Unblock Childhood Memories
This is a gentle essence that releases the fear that blocks childhood memories. Port Wine Magnolia allows these memories to be brought forward in a gentle way so that they can be dealt with and then let go of. This essence assists an adult in revisiting and opening up spiritual experiences obstructed since childhood.

FLE 46   Linden ♦ *Tilia cordata* 'Greenspire'
Release Chauvinism ♦ S
This essence is specially helpful for men. Linden releases the pattern of "male chauvinism"—being authoritarian, domineering, controlling, or insensitive in intimate relationships with females. It allows men to feel more sensitive and caring.

FLE 47   Purple Tulip Magnolia ✦ *Magnolia liliflora* 'Nigra'
Spirituality ✦ S

Purple Tulip Magnolia releases fear-based or controlling religious programming. It allows the natural spirituality of a person to emerge over time. This may or may not take an external form such as a religion or a philosophy.

FLE 48   Davy Filbert ✦ *Corylus avellana* 'Daviana'
Physical Self-Image ✦ M

Davy Filbert is for those who are obsessive about improving their physical appearance with makeup, beauty treatments, cosmetic surgery, exercise programs, dieting, and so forth. The essence releases the underlying self-rejection that drives this obsession. It allows the person to make choices about whether to pursue these options rather than being driven by a strong sense of physical inadequacy.

FLE 49   Purple Weeping Japanese Maple ✦ *Acer palmatum* 'Dissectum Atropurpureum'
Perfectionism ✦ M

The essence of this variety of Japanese maple is for the perfectionist who is under the continual stress of achieving superhuman results in life. The essence releases the unrealistic expectations from the conscious and subconscious mind. The person can then delight in simply being a fallible human being who makes a mistake every now and then.

FLE 50   Bush Cherry ✦ *Prunus glandulosa*
Tumors ✦ M

Bush Cherry is for treating tumors. It can be used to assist in tumor size reduction; it targets abnormal, premalignant, and malignant tissues and helps weaken and break down such tissue. It also assists in eliminating the toxins that result from tumor reduction. Taking Bush

Cherry does not clash with conventional cancer treatments such as chemotherapy and radiotherapy. The typical dose is 5 drops three times daily.

FLE 51   Mexican Hawthorn ✦ *Crataegus pubescens*
Death

Mexican Hawthorn is for the person who is facing death. It helps promote acceptance by assisting in releasing the fear of death and supports the gentle letting go of the need to stay for others. This essence can be used for actual physical death but also for the death experience of leaving a job, a house, or a relationship after a long period of time.

FLE 52   White Fringe Tree ✦ *Chionanthus virginicus*
Chest ✦ P

White Fringe Tree is excellent for upper respiratory tract infections, bronchitis, some influenza, pneumonia, pleurisy, and the common cold. It may cause the virus and/or the bacterium to be released through the natural body fluids, and it may help prevent secondary complications. However, for potentially serious chest infections, the essence should be considered an adjunct, not an alternative, to conventional medical treatment.

FLE 53   Crab Apple ✦ *Malus ioensis*
Elixir of Youth ✦ S

Crab Apple lessens a person's emotional and mental difficulties that may have worn him or her down, opens the mind and emotions to new possibilities, and gives a new zest for life. It restores one's vigor for life on every level. It is appropriate for those who are experiencing a stagnation in life that constantly inhibits them from extending themselves into new areas.

FLE 54   Sugar Maple ♦ *Acer saccharum*
Veins/Capillaries ♦ P

This essence promotes better circulation through surface (varicose) veins and capillaries. For best results, also supplement the diet with antioxidant vitamins (A, C, and E) and bioflavonoids. In the mental realm, Sugar Maple assists with bringing to a person's awareness the mental and/or emotional restrictions that have possibly allowed this circulatory imbalance to develop.

FLE 55   Simon's Poplar ♦ *Populus simonii* 'Fastigiata'
Arteries and Veins ♦ P

Simon's Poplar assists in reducing fat deposits in veins and arteries; therefore, it is of use in the early stages of atherosclerosis. It is a good adjunct to Sugar Maple (FLE 54). Simon's Poplar particularly addresses the emotional imbalances that contribute to artery and vein problems. See essence Holm Oak (FLE 147) as well.

FLE 56   Dutch Elm ♦ *Ulmus* x *hollandica*
Mental Functions ♦ M

Dutch Elm encourages mental clarity and memory retention. Dutch Elm affects both short-term and long-term memory and assists those people who find that they often experience fuzzy or confused mental thought processes. It brings a clearer, sharper focus to thinking. It possibly could be of some use in treating Alzheimer's disease, dementia, manic depression, and schizophrenia.

FLE 57   Persimmon ♦ *Diospiros kaki*
Release Home ♦ S

Persimmon helps a person release and neutralize ties to an old home and open up to a new experience. It applies especially to people who leave a home they have had for a long time (for example, to go into a nursing or retirement home). It can assist people in becoming comfortable in their new environment.

FLE 58   Lily-of-the-Valley Tree ✦ *Clethra arborea*
Malignancy ✦ S

This essence will help release and neutralize fear of an existing malignancy, balancing the emotions to enable an opening up to new possibilities of what this malignancy may bring into a person's life. It brings awareness on a spiritual level of the imbalance that exists in the person's life. It also brings a sense of detachment from the situation, enough to allow the person the space to deal with the whole complex situation, giving him or her the ability to assess what is the best approach to treatment.

FLE 59   Pomegranate ✦ *Punica granatum*
After Stroke

In the physical realm, this essence may assist damaged brain cells and tissue and help in recovering the use of impaired functions, to the extent that this is possible. In the emotional realm, it will increase openness and help release fear and frustration. In the mental realm, it will help release negative thought patterns and open the way to a more positive attitude.

FLE 60   Callery Pear ✦ *Pyrus calleryana*
Eyes ✦ M

Callery Pear removes the proverbial rose-colored glasses and helps the person to see people (and things) as they really are. It assists a person who for a long time has been immersed in a situation in which he or she has had no clarity or ability to see the reality.

FLE 61   Cut-leaf Norway Maple (Sherbrooke) ✦
Acer platanoides 'Lorbergii'
Skin, Ears, Nose, Throat ✦ P

This essence works on the endocrine glands, which control the flora of those places where bacteria may enter the body: the skin, ears, nose, and throat. Symptoms that may be addressed include watery or dry eyes, dry or sore throat, earache, excessive or insufficient ear-wax production, hay fever, eczema, rash, and hives. This essence may assist acne, body odor, boils, chicken pox, cold sores, deafness, encephalitis, foot odor, German measles, hearing problems, herpes, loss of smell, loss of taste, measles, Menière's disease, mumps, psoriasis, shingles, skin scar tissue, and tonsillitis. In the emotional realm, Norway Maple FLE 61 brings to the person's awareness the things in his or her life that hold some irritation.

FLE 62   Flowering Peach ✦ *Prunus persica* cv.
Prostate ✦ P

This essence will work in the physical realm in respect to all types of prostate problems by balancing and releasing toxins. It can be helpful in cases of impotence. The use of Flowering Peach is also appropriate before and after prostate surgery. It may increase sperm count. It is a companion essence to FLE 140, Bleeding Heart Tree, which has a toning and strengthening effect on the prostate.

FLE 63   Red Cedar ✦ *Toona ciliata*
Injury ✦ P

Red Cedar works by sending energy and blood to the injured body part. It can help alleviate effects of shock and also help heal injuries in the elderly or in diabetics. In cases where the injury is not recent, this essence still applies. It should be taken orally and it may also be applied externally to the injured area as drops or a cream. It may help bunions, leg abscesses, and surface injuries.

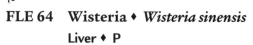

FLE 64   Wisteria ♦ *Wisteria sinensis*
Liver ♦ P

Wisteria can assist in the release and neutralizing of toxins and in balancing the functions of the liver. High cholesterol, gallbladder failure, hepatitis (A, B, C, D, E, and F), cirrhosis, liver failure, and jaundice may all be assisted by this essence. Wisteria is also very useful in correcting more subtle but real imbalances of the liver that are not advanced enough to show up in standard blood tests.

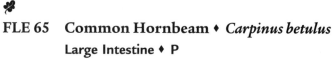

FLE 65   Common Hornbeam ♦ *Carpinus betulus*
Large Intestine ♦ P

Common Hornbeam works by balancing digestion and bacterial flora in the large intestine. It may assist chronic diarrhea, constipation (flaccid, spastic, and diverticulitis), hemorrhoids, and irritable bowel syndrome. In the emotional realm, if the person seeks awareness around this imbalance, Common Hornbeam brings understanding.

FLE 66   Pussy Willow (Goat Willow) ♦ *Salix x reichardtii*
Back ♦ P

Pussy Willow is the classic essence for strains and sprains of the back and related muscular systems. It is helpful for back problems caused by wear and tear, such as "nurse's back," disk degeneration, sciatica, and lumbago. The essence catalyzes significant tissue repair and regeneration.

FLE 67   Tupelo ♦ *Nyssa sylvatica*
Headache ♦ P

Tupelo provides temporary relief from chronic headache, tension headache, and migraine. It is typically given at a dosage of 7 drops six times daily for an existing headache or 7 drops every half hour in the case of a headache that has just come on. This essence does not work deeply on underlying levels of causation, but it is helpful in releasing the existing symptom picture.

FLE 68   Sacred Yulan ✦ *Magnolia denudata*
Insomnia ✦ P

This essence works to help promote sleep by lowering the heart rate and slowing down the breathing to appropriate levels. In the mental realm, Sacred Yulan brings a calming effect to constant mental chatter, allowing the mind to relax.

FLE 69   Celtic Cascade ✦ *Salix* x *reichardtii* 'Pendula'
Nausea ✦ P

Celtic Cascade can be given for temporary relief from nausea. The essence works by releasing and neutralizing the cause of the nausea. It has a balancing effect on the stomach and liver. It is appropriate in cases of food poisoning (5 to 10 drops every 10 to 15 minutes) in conjunction with seeking medical advice.

FLE 70   Star Magnolia ✦ *Magnolia stellata*
Rheumatoid Arthritis ✦ P

Star Magnolia may assist in balancing energy in the joints, reducing the inflammation and deterioration of joint tissue associated with rheumatoid arthritis. It releases toxins and makes way for healthy tissue growth. It is helpful in easing pain and increasing mobility of joints. In the emotional realm, Star Magnolia assists in releasing the held-in emotions underlying this condition.

FLE 71   Peach ✦ *Prunus persica*
Personal Growth ✦ S

Personal growth can be one of the most challenging paths a person chooses to follow. Peach assists in the opening of the crown chakra and the third eye, which aids in spiritual growth. It may bring to a person's awareness specific aspects of the self that he or she may wish to address. It opens up a person to embracing inner changes.

FLE 72   White Flowering Plum ✦ *Prunus cerasifera* 'Pissardii'
Let Go of a Relationship ✦ S

White Flowering Plum releases emotional resentment and sadness, cleanses the mind, and prepares the person to start again. If the person is ready for emotional freedom, White Flowering Plum brings this to the situation. It is recommended for divorce and for the breakup of relationships, friendships, and business partnerships where there is a lot of ill-feeling.

FLE 73   Bradford Flowering Pear ✦
Pyrus calleryana 'Bradford'
Release Sadness ✦ M

This essence helps with the release of sadness of any kind, especially the "what might have been" feeling and the "knot in the stomach" feeling. It complements Dove Tree (FLE 3; Bereavement) and White Flowering Plum (FLE 72; Let Go of a Relationship).

FLE 74   American Nettle Tree (American Hackberry) ✦
Celtis occidentalis
Sinuses ✦ P

American Nettle Tree helps clear the sinuses—for example, in the case of chronic sinusitis, polyps, or hay fever. It promotes lymphatic drainage and nasal clearing of the sinuses in a strength proportional to the dosage used.

FLE 75   Camperdown Elm ✦ *Ulmus glabra* 'Camperdownii'
Osteoporosis ✦ P

This essence balances the body's absorption and retention of calcium. It may therefore be useful in the treatment and prevention of osteoporosis. It is helpful to use with English Elm (FLE 11) after menopause.

FLE 76   Chinese Michelia ♦ *Michelia doltsopa*
Pancreas ♦ P

This essence assists the pancreas primarily in balancing insulin production and to a lesser extent in producing digestive enzymes.

FLE 77   Trident Maple ♦ *Acer buergerianum*
Anxiety ♦ M

Trident Maple is recommended for anxiety, nervous tension, and unspecified fears caused by excessive mental activity. This essence will work in the mental and emotional realms to release the cause of the anxiety. It may help relieve physical symptoms associated with anxiety such as hyperventilation, palpitations, trembling, sweating, hot and cold flashes, dry throat, nausea, and headache.

FLE 78   Japanese Zelkova ♦ *Zelkova serrata*
Bladder Incontinence ♦ P

Japanese Zelkova helps strengthen the external sphincter muscle and related muscle groups, thereby helping bladder incontinence.

FLE 79   Black Oak ♦ *Quercus velutina*
Conjunctivitis ♦ P

Black Oak balances all eye fluids, neutralizing and releasing waste materials from them. It may assist in treating conjunctivitis, trachoma, glaucoma, and cataract formation. In the emotional and spiritual realms, Black Oak brings an awareness and understanding to the metaphysical reasons behind the eye imbalances.

FLE 80   European Pussy Willow ♦ *Salix discolor*
Depression ♦ S

European Pussy Willow is recommended for depression caused by excessive mental activity that results in a negative thought pattern. The essence will release and neutralize the negative thought pattern and provide balance. It will address mental and emotional problems like loss of interest, brooding, the "everything is too hard" feeling, "black cloud" syndrome, and the "what have I done to deserve this" feeling.

FLE 81   Japanese Maple ♦ *Acer palmatum*
Emphysema/Recurrent Chest Infection ♦ P

Japanese Maple revitalizes the air sacs (alveoli) at the ends of the bronchial tree branches. It may help with some regeneration of damaged air sacs in the lungs. It can be very useful in strengthening the lungs after recurrent chest infections.

This is a beautiful, gentle essence that soothes as its energy flows through the person's energy field, focusing particularly on the respiratory system. It brings with it the release of long-suppressed emotions, and it assists in reeducating the lungs on how to breathe fully again.

It is important to have realistic expectations when treating serious medical conditions such as emphysema using falling leaf essences. While some extent of improvement may be possible, to expect falling leaf essences to cure such a chronic degenerative condition is not realistic.

FLE 82   Flowering Ash (Manna Ash) ♦ *Fraxinus ornus*
Eyes—Deterioration ♦ P

Eyesight deterioration of any kind creates a certain level of stress that can be at times quite difficult to deal with. Flowering Ash may help correct any problems with the coatings (retina, cornea) and muscles (iris, pupils) of the eyes. It also assists in improving farsightedness, shortsightedness, astigmatism, and presbyopia ("old eyes").

FLE 83   Jacaranda ♦ *Jacaranda acutifolia*
Sex Drive ♦ M

Jacaranda balances the libido and may also address erectile dysfunction and ejaculatory impotence, frigidity, nymphomania, and satyriasis on a physical and emotional level. Sometimes imbalances in a person's sex drive are caused not by a physical problem but by a very potent emotional difficulty. Jacaranda seeks to assist with developing awareness and understanding of the underlying core issue of the sexual imbalance.

FLE 84   Cockspur Hawthorn ✦ *Crataegus crus-galli*
Snoring ✦ P

This essence assists with temporary or chronic snoring.

FLE 85   White Cedar ✦ *Melia azedarach* var. *australasica*
Hair Loss (Balding) ✦ P

White Cedar may assist the problem of hair loss regardless of its cause or the length of time that the condition has existed. (But be reasonable in your expectations of improvement.)

FLE 86   Spring Cherry (Weeping Rosebud Cherry) ✦ *Prunus pendula*
Cellulite ✦ P

Cellulite occurs when lymphatic drainage is not activated. Toxic waste is trapped in the skin and tissues become inflamed as a result. This essence may assist the drainage (opening and balancing the lymphatic system) and release trapped toxins.

Emotionally, Spring Cherry brings with it a new energy that allows the release of negative emotions that are blocking the movement of toxins represented by the cellulite. It is a bit like spring cleaning.

FLE 87   Japanese Maple ✦ *Acer palmatum* 'Omurayama'
Irritable Bowel ✦ P

This essence balances bowel bacteria and is particularly effective for treating an overgrowth of the yeast *Candida*. It works best with oral supplementation of normal bowel bacteria. "Die-off" of *Candida* or other inappropriately overrepresented bowel microorganisms can occur from about day 2 to day 20 of taking this essence. This die-off can temporarily exacerbate the symptoms.

FLE 88   Scotch Elm ✦ *Ulmus glabra*
Life Purpose
Scotch Elm resolves blocks to the intuitive perception of one's life purpose. Use for three to six months in stubborn cases. Ineffectiveness usually indicates the need for more resolution of emotional or mental blockages.

FLE 89   Golden Ash ✦ *Fraxinus excelsior* 'Aurea'
Metaphysical Awareness
To the extent that a person is ready for it, Golden Ash resolves blocks to metaphysical seeing and hearing. It is useful at an appropriate stage in spiritual growth.

FLE 90   Flowering Cherry ✦ *Prunus serrulata* 'Mt. Fuji'
Reflection ✦ S
Flowering Cherry encourages reflection and growth. The essence promotes a healthy introspective and reflective look at life. In this reflection on the past, lessons or learnings that are useful in both present and future become apparent.

FLE 91   Hedge Maple (Field Maple) ✦ *Acer campestre*
Release Disillusion ✦ M
All of us at some time in our lives have experienced disillusionment, but the important question is whether we move on from that point of disillusionment at the appropriate time. Hedge Maple brings to a person's consciousness the reasons that he or she has remained in this state of disillusionment and gives the impetus to move beyond this point with a new approach or perspective.

FLE 92   Manchurian Pear ✦ *Pyrus ussuriensis*
Release Grief ✦ S

Grief can be a paralyzing emotion. In tribal cultures, time and space were made through ritual to allow grieving people a way of expressing their emotions; the ritual honored those emotions. Such rituals accepted grief as a healing process and assisted in the gradual release of the emotion. When a person experiences grief through its various stages, he or she grows in maturity and wisdom. In today's society, we are not adequately equipped to deal with the grief experiences that are an integral part of life. When we are grieving, we just continue on with everyday life and do not give due credit to the grieving experience, often suppressing it and in some way causing on a soul level loss to our being. Manchurian Pear brings a more positive outcome by releasing the grief in stages.

FLE 93   Red Oak ✦ *Quercus rubra*
Release Bitterness ✦ M

Red Oak addresses the causal difficulty at a soul level that keeps a person holding onto bitterness. Like the emotion of hatred, bitterness can diminish a person's life force and block his or her life's purpose and full potential. If the person is willing, he or she can be confronted with the part he or she played in the situation that has created the bitterness and allowed it to endure. Once a person chooses to see this reality and what it is within the soul that would benefit from change, Red Oak will assist with releasing bitter emotions and at the same time bring strength to the person so that he or she can look at the situation in a new light.

FLE 94   Japanese Barberry 'Golden Ring' ✦
Berberis thunbergii 'Golden Ring'
Release Fear of Poverty ✦ M

Some of us are plagued by a fear of poverty, which can become all consuming. Many decisions we make can be influenced by this fear, consciously or unconsciously. If we looked at this objectively, we would see that continuing to make decisions based on a fear has an inhibiting effect on some very important things in our lives. Japanese Barberry 'Golden Ring' allows a golden ring to form energetically, dissolving the energy ties to the mind-set of poverty and allowing us to develop our own beliefs about abundance in our life.

FLE 95   Eastern Red Bud ✦ *Cercis canadensis*
Release Fear of Abandonment ✦ M

The fear of abandonment is a very real and often disempowering emotion. Many of us have in some way experienced it to some degree, most often in our childhood. If as an adult this fear continues and controls how we relate to others in our life, we can find that in many situations we are not responding as an adult, from a point of balance and inner strength. Eastern Red Bud seeks to assist with the release of fear of abandonment and brings with it the ability to make balanced choices.

FLE 96   Kilmarnock Willow ✦
Salix x *reichardtii* 'Kilmarnock'
Release Fear of Dependency ✦ M

Kilmarnock Willow assists us in seeing where we are overly independent in our life—that is, where we are stubborn and will not accept help when we require it. Fear of dependency can in many ways stop relationships from developing fully. When we fear dependency upon another, we tend to block the flow of giving and receiving between ourselves and those whom we relate to. This sets up a feeling of isolation. When we open up to accepting that we can receive help from others without losing our independence, we become more open to life's experiences.

FLE 97   Sorrell Tree (Sourwood) ✦ *Oxydendrum arboreum*
Release Fear of Imperfection ✦ M

We all seek to find that which lies deep within us—our own perfect self. The problem is that we look outside ourselves and see the (seeming) perfection of others and then try to emulate this, not realizing that what is perfect for one person is not necessarily perfect for another.

Fear of imperfection blocks each one of us from developing our full potential because it inhibits what we choose to do in our lives. Our greatest learning comes from our greatest mistakes. Sorrell Tree brings to our awareness the core issues around this fear of imperfection and assists us in seeing that we can make mistakes and still have a life and friends. This essence allows us to be real. (What a relief!)

FLE 98   Cypress Oak ♦ *Quercus robur* 'Fastigiata'
Release Fear of Dying

As children, most of us do not have a fear of death. This develops only as we become aware of our mortality and see that things have a cycle of birth and death. In many ways our fear develops because we are disconnected from spirit, and we do not believe in, or we doubt our belief in, an afterlife. Cypress Oak reconnects us to spirit in the form that is appropriate for each one of us. This connection helps us understand that there is something beyond death and supports each one of us when dealing with our own mortality and the mortality of others.

FLE 99   Snowball Tree (Guelder Rose) ♦ *Viburnum opulus*
Release Fear of Illness ♦ S

Our own illness or the illness of another can be a very challenging experience. When someone close to us becomes ill, we find that we need to get as far away from the situation as is possible. Fear often arises from a feeling of helplessness—there is nothing we can do to fix the person who is ill. Snowball Tree cushions the situation by bringing an understanding of this fear and the ability to see the bigger picture and the metaphysical insights surrounding the illness. It allows us to see that we all have our own journey, and while we may not be able to fix the ill person, we certainly can provide great support with love and care. From this point we can overcome our fear and be fully present for the ill person. This essence also addresses the person who is struggling with illness. It helps the person direct energy into healing, instead of into fear of the sickness.

FLE 100 Smokebush ◆ *Cotinus coggygria* 'Flame'

Release Fear of Disability ◆ M

Smokebush helps people who have had someone close to them become disabled and they have difficulty relating to this situation. This essence enables the fear of disability to be released and a more positive relationship to be established with the disabled person. It is recommended not only for family members but also for anyone closely associated with a disabled person.

FLE 101 Green Honey Locust ◆ *Gleditsia triacanthos* 'Shademaster'

Release Fear of Rejection ◆ M

Green Honey Locust addresses all situations in which a fear of rejection holds us back from our true pathway. Fear of rejection stops many relationships from developing into their full expression of love. We experience attraction to another person but stop short of really committing ourselves to the experience because we fear that the feeling may not be reciprocated. Of course, this is exactly what the other person has done also, which leads us to an impasse. Love is not the only arena in which fear of rejection blocks us from reaching our full potential. For instance, if we fear rejection, we may decide not to apply for a higher-paid job because we are afraid of being turned down.

FLE 102 Weeping Maple ◆ *Acer palmatum* 'Sekimori'

Release Fear of Inadequacy

In our modern society, we can be plagued by feelings of inadequacy because there is always a high standard to live up to. Weeping Maple brings to us a strong sense of self and a realization that whatever we do, we will do it to the best of our ability.

FLE 103 Young's Weeping Birch ✦ *Betula pendula* 'Youngii'
Release Fear of Happiness ✦ S

As human beings, our existence here on the earth consists of a constant search for happiness. However, in many situations we find ourselves doing things that sabotage happiness. Why would we do this? We may fear happiness because we fear losing that happiness. For some of us, this fear controls everything we do. Young's Weeping Birch assists us in understanding the core issue causing this fear and brings strength for us to face and let go of the fear, knowing that the cause is no longer relevant in our life.

FLE 104 Purple Leaf Pink Flowering Plum ✦ *Prunus cerasifera* 'Nigra'
Release Fear of Commitment ✦ S

All fears inhibit our life force in one way or another. Fear of commitment allows us to stay in a "safe" place, but always being safe does not allow us to experience what we came here to become on this earth. Purple Leaf Pink Flowering Plum addresses all situations in which a fear of commitment exists—relationships, career, sports and the required training, spiritual growth, and much more. In the case where a person lacks commitment to life in general, this essence works exceptionally well.

FLE 105 Ubame Oak ✦ *Quercus phillyraeoides*
Release Fear of Disappointment ✦ S

The fear of disappointment keeps high walls around those who allow it to manifest in their life. We all experience disappointment at some time, but it is how we respond to the situation that assists us in moving beyond the disappointment into awareness and understanding. If we expect to be disappointed, it is most likely that we will be. But once we are able to release the fear of disappointment, we become freer and much more willing to taste the richness of life's experience, with all its ups and downs.

FLE 106 Cut-leaf Birch ✦ *Betula pendula* 'Dalecarlica'
Release Fear of Loss ✦ M

Many of our experiences in life involve loss. We lose to the boy down the road in a bike race, the swimming race we trained so hard for was lost to a stronger swimmer, and the important job we applied for has been given to another applicant. This is all a part of life. Fear of losing will stop us from participating in the beneficial opportunities presented to us. But it is in this experience of loss that we find better ways of doing things and we become more determined, stronger, more polished. In a way each loss, if used positively, can be built on to create a better life all around. Cut-leaf Birch assists with releasing the fear of losing so that we can participate fully in life's opportunities.

FLE 107 Lilac ✦ *Syringa* x *hyacinthiflora*
Release Detachment ✦ S

Detachment can sometimes serve a person well, but constant detachment from life can cause very serious problems. When we are perpetually detached, we find that we are not really in touch with the people in our life; relationships, career, and creativity all suffer. Lilac assists the detached person in becoming more involved in life, helping the person see the unity of all people and all of nature.

FLE 108 Magnolia 'Alexandrina' ✦
Magnolia x *soulangeana* 'Alexandrina'
Release Fear of Aging ✦ M

In today's constant media coverage of the "beautiful people" of the world, it is not hard to understand why many people struggle with the fear of aging; we are always exposed to the ideal image of the perfect woman or man. If we allowed this to run our life, we would be always seeking the newest innovation to keep ourselves forever young. A lot of energy goes into the maintaining of an image. This essence assists in the release of the fear of aging and allows us to see beyond surface beauty to the real inner beauty within us all. It strongly addresses the emotional realm.

FLE 109 White Flowering Dogwood ♦ *Cornus florida* 'Alba'
Release Fear of "Losing Face" ♦ M

Pride can create difficulties in our lives on many levels. The fear of "losing face" takes us into situations where we cannot necessarily cope to the best of our ability but, instead of enlisting help, struggle on regardless. White Flowering Dogwood brings to us an awareness of the situations in which we are not facing reality and shows us why we are not being true to ourselves.

FLE 110 Golden Locust ♦ *Robinia pseudoacacia* 'Frisia'
Release Fear of Loneliness ♦ S

At certain points in our lives we may be lonely. There can be many reasons for this, whether we have just ended a relationship, have lost touch with our friends, have just moved to a new town, or have just taken on a new job. At these times there appears to be no one there for us. A fear of loneliness can keep us locked in a situation that is no longer right purely because we fear to leave what is comfortable. Golden Locust allows these feelings to come to the surface and then brings to our awareness the connection we have with all things. It encourages the ability to be comfortable while being alone and allows us to see that when we are alone, we have our deepest insights into life. We realize that lack of human companionship does not mean that we are alone. This essence allows us to connect fully to spirit.

FLE 111 Burr Oak (Mossy Cup Oak) ♦ *Quercus macrocarpa*
Release Fear of Inadequacy ♦ M

One of the most difficult fears to handle is the fear of inadequacy. In the worst-case scenario, it can affect almost every aspect of our life. On a lesser scale, it can be specific to a certain aspect of our life. Burr Oak helps us understand the issues that allow this fear to manifest.

In reality, our ability in any given situation may well meet and exceed the demands of the situation, but if we fear being seen as inadequate, we may not attempt or strive to finish a task or challenge. This essence helps us release the fear of inadequacy, thereby allowing new doors to open in our lives.

FLE 112 Canoe Birch ✦ *Betula papyrifera*
Release Greed ✦ S

Our culture today focuses on the constant acquisition of material wealth, often to the detriment of our emotional, mental, and spiritual wealth. This material intensity is healthy if it is in balance, but sometimes it can manifest in our lives as greed, which leads to an unhappy way of being. Energetically it blocks the flow of energy—the giving and receiving—in our existence. Greed springs from an underlying belief that the world lacks enough for all its inhabitants. Canoe Birch brings understanding to those of us who are willing to release greed in our lives and assists us in changing this difficult imbalance. In the United States Canoe Birch is known as White Birch.

FLE 113 Wintersweet (Allspice) ✦ *Chimonanthus praecox*
Release Dependency ✦ S

Dependency of any kind is limiting to both the person who is dependant and the person upon whom one is dependent. It stops individualization and the journeying along one's own pathway in life. In a way, it prevents both parties from achieving their full potential and can set up resentment between the parties involved. Wintersweet helps both parties emerge from such a dysfunctional dependency.

FLE 114 Crazy Filbert ✦ *Corylus avellana* 'Contorta'
Release Dislike ✦ M

As with all difficult emotions, disliking someone, something, or a situation keeps us energetically tied into a constant cycle that serves no constructive purpose. To work with this emotion and release it allows a freeing up of our energy so that it can be put to better use. Crazy

Filbert assists us in releasing a dislike and helps us see that there is no need to hold on to emotion. The essence also brings us understanding of the underlying emotion that may create this dislike.

FLE 115 Pagoda Tree ♦ *Sophora japonica* 'Pendula'
Release Revenge ♦ S

Revenge can be a very consuming and debilitating intention that demands a lot of destructive energy. Revenge brings out the worst in human nature. When a person who is dealing with the desire for revenge finally realizes the destructiveness of his or her intentions and chooses to release them, his or her whole focus on life can change. Pagoda Tree brings with it a fresh, cleansing energy and dissolves the tight knots that bind the person caught up in the energy of revenge.

FLE 116 Golden Italian Poplar ♦
Populus x *canadensis* 'Serotina Aurea'
Release Intolerance ♦ M

Intolerance is often born out of lack of understanding or empathy for a situation. It can also exist as an aspect of a person's way of relating to other people because he or she is unable to see things from another's perspective. Golden Italian Poplar brings to the person the ability to empathize with others and to see that everyone has his or her own way of being. It brings acceptance of others.

FLE 117 Dawn Redwood ♦ *Metasequoia glyptostroboides*
Release Hypersensitivity ♦ M

Dawn Redwood releases a pattern of hypersensitivity to life in the mental realm. It helps those who tend to overreact to seemingly small events or small issues. The essence resolves underlying stress to produce a calmer disposition, a greater mental stamina, and resistance to external stresses. This in turn calms the emotions.

FLE 118 Cut-leaf Norway Maple (Emerald) ◆
Acer platanoides 'Lorbergii'
Release "Life Is Hard" ◆ M

This essence releases the belief that life is difficult. It allows one to move beyond the self-sabotage that is necessary to maintain this belief into a life of flow, abundance, and meaning. This essence is similar to FLE 31 Silver Birch, but it is deeper in its action. Whereas FLE 31 is most useful for bringing about subconscious, perceptual change, FLE 118 works more on the level of promoting positive action in the here and now. Both essences can be given simultaneously in stubborn cases.

> Note that FLE 118, like FLE 61, is also Cut-leaf Norway Maple. Although the action of essences made from leaves collected from the same plant in different locations is usually the same, occasionally it is quite different. FLE 61 and FLE 118 offer an example of essences collected from trees that are the same in type but come from different locations and are distinctly different in action.

FLE 119 Maybush (Reeve's Spirea) ◆ *Spirea cantoniensis*
Female Self-Confidence

Maybush is recommended primarily for helping women with issues of self-esteem and self-confidence. It releases from the subconscious the idea that women are somehow inferior to men, or less competent than men, or incapable of independent living, or of less value in a "man's world." It results in more powerful, confident living for women.

FLE 120 Maidenhair Tree ◆ *Ginkgo biloba*
Release Inconsideration of Others ◆ S

Maidenhair Tree releases a pattern of being insufficiently considerate of others in interpersonal relationships. This results in empathy and a clear appreciation of others' feelings and perspective.

FLE 121 Weeping Maple ✦ *Acer palmatum* 'Red Filigree Lace'
Lateral Thinking ✦ M

This essence releases programmed boundaries to thought processes. In resolving these educationally induced blockages, the essence takes one out of thinking in "boxes" into an understanding of the interrelatedness of all life on all levels. It facilitates lateral, creative thinking and promotes ongoing evaluation and questioning of long-held beliefs.

FLE 122 White Horse Chestnut ✦ *Aesculus hippocastanum*
Assists Kundalini

White Horse Chestnut releases resistance in the mental realm to kundalini and the changes that ensue from it. It may be given to alleviate the numerous distressing symptoms from the movement of kundalini, which are usually symptoms of resistance. It may also be given for up to two years after kundalini abates to help integrate the massive changes that the energy can bring.

FLE 123 Weeping Mulberry ✦ *Morus* sp.
Unites Thought and Feeling ✦ M

Weeping Mulberry removes boundaries between thought and feeling. It enables one to move beyond either primarily thinking or primarily feeling, or thinking and feeling simultaneously but disharmoniously. This essence releases the switch between thought and feeling so that these aspects can coexist harmoniously in unity.

FLE 124 Spice Bush (Californian Allspice) ✦
Calycanthus occidentalis
Obsessive Behaviors ✦ M

Spice Bush is recommended for obsessive, compulsive behaviors other than substance addiction. This essence helps release underlying needs for the compulsive behavior. The typical dosage is 4 drops three times daily. It is generally used for more serious, chronic cases.

FLE 125 Linden ✦ *Tilia dasystyla*
Minor Substance Addiction ✦ M

For minor substance addiction, such as to caffeine, chocolate, or sugar, 7 drops of Linden twice daily will help. This essence releases mental and emotional dependency.

FLE 126 Oriental Liquidamber ✦ *Liquidambar orientalis*
Release Mental Reactivity ✦ M

Being mentally reactive to life stresses multiplies the stress. For example, if one becomes sick, one can work a lot of mental overtime worrying over how long the sickness will last and what the outcome will be. Of course, it is easier to recover from the sickness if one can relax and trust through the experience. Oriental Liquidamber helps release that pattern of reactivity to stress. It is a companion essence to Dawn Redwood (FLE 117), which applies to an overwrought nervous system.

FLE 127 Burning Bush ✦ *Euonymus alatus* 'Compactus'
Release Blame of Family ✦ S

Burning Bush releases the belief that the system or family is to blame for one's problems in life. In removing this projection, the essence brings one face-to-face with personal responsibility. It reveals one's path in life and the certainty of knowing that it is only oneself who can follow or block this path. It is excellent for releasing the convict or victim mentality from the subconscious mind.

FLE 128 Korean Viburnum ✦ *Viburnum carlesii*
Perception of Aging ✦ M

The notion that aging is a negative experience and that older people, particularly women, are intrinsically of less value to society is not strange. Korean Viburnum releases that perception. In this regard the essence is excellent in addressing the mental perceptions and cultural programming that can underlie or accompany menopausal problems.

FLE 129 Chinese Witch Hazel ♦ *Hamamelis mollis*
Release "Busyness" ♦ M

Chinese Witch Hazel releases the mental programming that says one must be continually busy to be okay. It allows one to stop, have a cup of tea, sniff the roses, and daydream for a while—all without appreciable guilt.

FLE 130 Turkistan Birch ♦ *Betula ? turkistanica*
Release Persistent Anxiety ♦ M

To release the mental thought patterns that underlie persistent anxiety, Turkistan Birch is excellent. It addresses the type of persistent anxiety that manifests in the emotional realm but is continually generated by thought patterns at the mental level—worry, pessimism, recurrent doubts, and so on.

FLE 131 Kentucky Coffee Tree ♦ *Gymnocladus dioica*
Acceptance of Body ♦ S

Kentucky Coffee Tree is recommended for the physically self-conscious and those who find difficulty in fully accepting the height, weight, contour, or appearance of their physical body. It releases the tendency to compare one's body with some hypothetical "ideal" body, against which it is judged to be inferior or inadequate. The result is an acceptance and appreciation of one's physical self.

FLE 132 Spiked Winter Hazel ♦ *Corylopsis spicata*
Peer Group Pressure ♦ M

This essence releases the need for acceptance and approval by the peer group. It is recommended for those who find that this need leads them to behave in a group in a way contrary to their own nature.

FLE 133 Hornbeam ♦ *Carpinus betulus* 'Fastigiata'
Release Superiority ♦ S

Hornbeam releases the need to consider oneself superior to others spiritually, mentally, or emotionally. Underlying this need is low self-esteem, stemming usually from a difficult childhood or some form of early abuse.

FLE 134 Golden Elm ♦ *Ulmus procera* 'Louis van Houtte'
Lesser Obsessive Behaviors ♦ M

Golden Elm is recommended for lesser cases of obsessive behavior. It releases patterns of time-wasting by overabsorption in a particular habitual pursuit, such as watching television, surfing the Internet, or talking on the telephone. Thus, it helps restore a better pattern of life balance.

For more serious cases of obsessive, compulsive behavior, see Spice Bush (FLE 124).

FLE 135 Flowering Dogwood ♦ *Cornus florida*
Life Balance

This essence is for those who tend to be obsessive or to overemphasize a particular area of life at the expense of life balance overall. It releases the need to preserve the imbalance so that a better balance can emerge.

FLE 136 Box Elder (Ghost Maple) ♦ *Acer negundo*
Value Emotions ♦ M

Box Elder releases the belief that the realm of thought (reason, intellect) is more important or more reliable than the realm of feeling or emotion. It is excellent for those who ignore or abuse their emotional realm.

FLE 137 Flowering Almond 'Double Crimson' ♦
Prunus dulcis 'Double Crimson'
Dental Pain ♦ P

This essence is useful for tooth and gum pain. For short-term relief take 7 drops every hour or even more frequently, as required. Taken at 7 drops twice daily over a longer period, the essence has a strengthening, toning, and detoxifying effect on gum tissue. It is capable of dealing with gum and tooth infection to a certain extent, although it is no substitute for a dentist if pain persists.

FLE 138 African Laburnum ♦ *Calpurnia aurea*
Skin Problems ♦ P

This essence is generally applicable to skin problems, including acne, dermatitis, and eczema. It releases toxicity from the liver, lymphatic system, and skin. In the emotional realm, African Laburnum grants understanding of the problem to the affected person.

FLE 139 David's Snake Bark Maple ♦ *Acer davidii*
Serious Viral Infection ♦ P

This essence can assist in the treatment of HIV and other serious chronic viral infections such as Epstein-Barr and glandular fever. It may be applicable at any stage of the disease. The typical dosage is 5 drops four times daily. It helps people mentally release negative thought patterns and physically release the toxins from viruses and other infections.

FLE 140 Bleeding Heart Tree ♦ *Omalanthus populifolius*
Prostate ♦ P

Bleeding Heart Tree taken 5 drops twice daily tones and strengthens the prostate, especially in men over 60 years of age. At 5 drops four times daily, it a useful treatment for cancer of the prostate (but is not a substitute for other established forms of treatment). In cases involving serious prostate problems, consider Flowering Peach (FLE 62).

FLE 141 Silver Linden ✦ *Tilia tomentosa*
Wound Healing ✦ P

Silver Linden facilitates healing of deep wounds or breakages in connective tissue or bone. It helps bond stressed or cleaved tissues and accelerates the healing process. It should be given orally only.

FLE 142 Indian Bean Tree ✦ *Catalpa bignonioides*
Foot Problems ✦ P

This essence is excellent for the healing of a variety of problems of the feet, including blisters, bruises, tinea, toenail problems, fractures, soreness, and swelling.

FLE 143 Snowy Mespilus ✦ *Amelanchier canadensis*
Infertility ✦ S

This essence can help treat infertility without discernible cause. Women should take it for up to six months. It also useful for men in cases of low sperm count or poor motility over a similar time frame.

FLE 144 Snake Bark (Manchustriped Maple) ✦
Acer tegmentosum
Blood Pressure ✦ P

Snake Bark balances the entire circulatory system and is used to assist in the treatment of high blood pressure. For chronic high blood pressure, continue treatment for three to six months. The essence can be taken even if pharmaceutical treatment is also followed.

FLE 145 Silver Pear ✦ *Pyrus salicifolia*
Chronic Viral Infections ✦ P

Silver Pear is helpful for treating chronic viral infections such as chronic fatigue syndrome. Physically, this essence promotes the elimination of viruses. Mentally, it releases the notion of the viral infection being powerful, promoting a subconscious belief that the immune system is sufficient to meet the challenge. It can also be given for more serious, persistent influenza. See also David's Snake Bark Maple (FLE 139).

FLE 146 Weeping Mulberry ✦ *Morus alba* 'Pendula'
Varicose Veins ✦ P

Weeping Mulberry can decrease varicose veins by improving the tone and strength of the vein walls. In stubborn cases, the essence must be taken for three to six months. This essence is for particularly difficult cases that do not respond to lesser treatment, such as with Sugar Maple (FLE 54), or to bring further improvement when other essences or treatments have exhausted their benefit.

FLE 147 Holm Oak ✦ *Quercus ilex*
Vascular Cleansing ✦ P

Holm Oak has a strong cleansing action on the walls of arteries, veins, and capillaries. It works much more deeply and strongly than Simon's Poplar (FLE 55), which it usually follows. The typical dosage is 5 drops twice daily for up to four months. It should be remembered that such an essence, while useful for early-stage artery and vein wall deposits, is no substitute for more radical treatments in more advanced cases.

FLE 148 Judas Tree ✦ *Cercis siliquastrum*
Lymphatic Cleansing ✦ P

Judas Tree is a very powerful lymphatic cleanser that is usually given for three to ten weeks at a time. This essence is a very useful part of a cleansing or detoxification program.

FLE 149 Valley Oak ✦ *Quercus lobata*
Arm Problems ✦ P

Valley Oak can assist in the treatment of strains, sprains, bruises, skin problems, and other difficulties of the arms and hands.

FLE 150 Scarlet Oak ♦ *Quercus coccinea*
Shoulder Problems ♦ P

Scarlet Oak can assist in the treatment of joint pain, "frozen" shoulder, and bony and soft-tissue injuries in the shoulder area.

FLE 151 Liquidamber (Kallista) ♦ *Liquidambar styraciflua*
Group Harmony ♦ S

The Liquidamber falling leaf essence collected from Kallista releases limitations that people develop emotionally when they work in close quarters with others. It allows people to focus on their work while remaining in harmony with coworkers.

FLE 152 Chinese Wax Ash ♦ *Fraxinus chinensis*
Spiritual Connection ♦ S

Chinese Wax Ash releases the fear of spiritual reconnection at the heart level and assists us in opening our heart to the light. This essence helps heal and release heart wounds, in which we have closed down our heart and keep a tight control on being open to love and spiritual connection. It releases the need to keep our heart closed and dispels the darkness of traumas.

FLE 153 Horizontal Elm ♦ *Ulmus glabra* 'Horizontalis'
Expanded Perspective ♦ M

This essence helps one release a limited view of a certain situation and allows a broader expanse to become obvious. It also assists one in embracing other valid perspectives around a situation.

FLE 154 Photinia (Christmas Berry) ♦ *Photina beauverdiana*
Focus ♦ M

Photinia releases the need to scatter one's energy, bringing focus and centering.

FLE 155 American Smoke Tree ♦ *Cotinus obovatus*
Release Racism ♦ S

This essence releases the programmed racial discrimination that can be found in some people—even when they are not conscious of it. They may be dealing with these programmed feelings by avoiding situations that bring them face-to-face with the reality that they do, in fact, hold some form of racial discrimination.

FLE 156 Wheatley Elm (Jersey Elm) ♦ *Ulmus minor* 'Sarniensis'
Release Pain of Separation ♦ S

This essence releases the pain one experiences when a relationship breaks down. It can be particularly helpful for those who after such a change in their lives find that they still haven't let go of the relationship and are in a deep depression about this loss. This essence releases the deep pain and allows new energy to come in to the heart and soul. It offers love of the self, which enables new relationships to develop. See also White Flowering Plum (FLE 72).

FLE 157 Viburnum ♦ *Viburnum sieboldii*
Inner Confidence ♦ M

Viburnum releases the need to prove ourselves to others. It helps us see the part we play in our own lives and other peoples' lives and allows us to become more balanced when relating to others, whether it be family, work, or social situations.

FLE 158 Leatherwood ♦ *Cyrilla racemiflora*
Patience ♦ M

Leatherwood releases the need to rush things and allows one to see the merit in quietly pulling back and waiting.

FLE 159 Autumn Zephyr-Lily (Flower of the West Wind) ♦
Zephyranthes candida
Release Programmed Sexuality ♦ S

This essence releases the need to hold on to cultural or family programming around sexuality. It allows people to experience their true sexual nature, taking them into a more expressive, exotic expansion of sexuality, but with the awareness that what they feel is appropriate and in a sense pure for them.

FLE 160 Full Moon Maple ♦ *Acer japonicum*
Emotional Awareness

This essence expands one's capacity to feel into a situation. It allows an easier emotional pathway through the situation, enabling one to deal better with it in the mental and physical realms and to be spiritually more in tune with the circumstances.

In the physical realm, this essence is particularly good for constipation and hemorrhoids. It assists one in releasing the need to control.

Full Moon Maple also enhances other essences in the falling leaf range. It is the essence that opens the doorway or clears deep unconscious blocks so that the subsequent essences taken have a quicker, more effective result.

TABLE 5.1: ABBREVIATED DESCRIPTION OF THE
ACTIONS OF THE 160 FALLING LEAF ESSENCES

No.	Common Name	Primary Area of Essence Action
1	Claret Ash	Influenza
2	Linden	Tonic
3	Dove Tree	Bereavement
4	Turkey Oak	Endocrine System
5	Weeping Willow	Kidneys
6	English Hawthorn	Stomach and Pancreas
7	Cherry Plum	Emotional Well-being
8	Pin Oak	Fatigue
9	White Ash	Osteoarthritis
10	Liquidamber (Donvale)	Inflammation
11	English Elm	Female Reproductive System
12	Willow Pattern Tree (Golden Rain Tree)	Nervous Insomnia
13	Pink Horse Chestnut	Fluid Retention
14	Apricot	Release Anger
15	Domestic Fig	Release Guilt
16	Oriental Plane	Release Fear of Change
17	Weeping Katsura Tree	Release Fear of Love
18	Copper Beech	Release Hatred
19	Yellow Flowering Currant (Golden Currant)	Self-Esteem
20	Winter Hazel	Release Programmed Living
21	Lombardy Poplar	Substance Addiction
22	Glory Vine	Release Mental Control
23	Black Pussy Willow	Specific Low Self-Esteem
24	Sawtooth Oak (Bristle-tipped Oak)	"Stiff Upper Lip"
25	Elderberry	Sexuality
26	Tulip Tree	Heart
27	Persian Witch Hazel (Persian Ironwood)	Release Children
28	Rowan	After Surgery
29	Yeddo Cherry	Mental Flexibility
30	White Mulberry	Muscular Weakness
31	Silver Birch	Release Struggle
32	Silver Maple	Breasts
33	Japanese Dogwood	Gout
34	Plane Tree	Indigestion
35	Thornless Scarlet Honey Locust	Release Disappointment
36	Japanese White Birch	Release Envy
37	Thornless Golden Honey Locust	Release Jealousy
38	Red Crepe Myrtle	Release Possessiveness
39	Aspen	Release Loneliness

No.	Common Name	Primary Area of Essence Action
40	Chinese Trumpet Vine	Release Fear of the Unknown
41	Crepe Myrtle	Release Uncertainty
42	Red Maple (Canadian Maple)	Release Fear of Lack of Love
43	Chinese Elm	Release Inappropriate Individualism
44	Weeping Elm	Release Emotional Turmoil
45	Port Wine Magnolia	Unblock Childhood Memories
46	Linden	Release Chauvinism
47	Purple Tulip Magnolia	Spirituality
48	Davy Filbert	Physical Self-Image
49	Purple Weeping Japanese Maple	Perfectionism
50	Bush Cherry	Tumors
51	Mexican Hawthorn	Death
52	White Fringe Tree	Chest
53	Crab Apple	Elixir of Youth
54	Sugar Maple	Veins/Capillaries
55	Simon's Poplar	Arteries and Veins
56	Dutch Elm	Mental Functions
57	Persimmon	Release Home
58	Lily-of-the-Valley Tree	Malignancy
59	Pomegranate	After Stroke
60	Callery Pear	Eyes
61	Cut-leaf Norway Maple (Sherbrooke)	Skin, Ears, Nose, Throat
62	Flowering Peach	Prostate
63	Red Cedar	Injury
64	Wisteria	Liver
65	Common Hornbeam	Large Intestine
66	Pussy Willow (Goat Willow)	Back
67	Tupelo	Headache
68	Sacred Yulan	Insomnia
69	Celtic Cascade	Nausea
70	Star Magnolia	Rheumatoid Arthritis
71	Peach	Personal Growth
72	White Flowering Plum	Let Go of a Relationship
73	Bradford Flowering Pear	Release Sadness
74	American Nettle Tree (American Hackberry)	Sinuses
75	Camperdown Elm	Osteoporosis
76	Chinese Michelia	Pancreas
77	Trident Maple	Anxiety
78	Japanese Zelkova	Bladder Incontinence
79	Black Oak	Conjunctivitis
80	European Pussy Willow	Depression

No.	Common Name	Primary Area of Essence Action
81	Japanese Maple	Emphysema/Recurrent Chest Infection
82	Flowering Ash (Manna Ash)	Eyes—Deterioration
83	Jacaranda	Sex Drive
84	Cockspur Hawthorn	Snoring
85	White Cedar	Hair Loss (Balding)
86	Spring Cherry (Weeping Rosebud Cherry)	Cellulite
87	Japanese Maple	Irritable Bowel
88	Scotch Elm	Life Purpose
89	Golden Ash	Metaphysical Awareness
90	Flowering Cherry	Reflection
91	Hedge Maple (Field Maple)	Release Disillusion
92	Manchurian Pear	Release Grief
93	Red Oak	Release Bitterness
94	Japanese Barberry 'Golden Ring'	Release Fear of Poverty
95	Eastern Red Bud	Release Fear of Abandonment
96	Kilmarnock Willow	Release Fear of Dependency
97	Sorrell Tree (Sourwood)	Release Fear of Imperfection
98	Cypress Oak	Release Fear of Dying
99	Snowball Tree (Guelder Rose)	Release Fear of Illness
100	Smokebush	Release Fear of Disability
101	Green Honey Locust	Release Fear of Rejection
102	Weeping Maple	Release Inadequacy
103	Young's Weeping Birch	Release Fear of Happiness
104	Purple Leaf Pink Flowering Plum	Release Fear of Commitment
105	Ubame Oak	Release Fear of Disappointment
106	Cut-leaf Birch	Release Fear of Loss
107	Lilac	Release Detachment
108	Magnolia 'Alexandrina'	Release Fear of Aging
109	White Flowering Dogwood	Release Fear of Losing Face
110	Golden Locust	Release Fear of Loneliness
111	Burr Oak (Mossy Cup Oak)	Release Fear of Inadequacy
112	Canoe Birch	Release Greed
113	Wintersweet (Allspice)	Release Dependency
114	Crazy Filbert	Release Dislike
115	Pagoda Tree	Release Revenge
116	Golden Italian Poplar	Release Intolerance
117	Dawn Redwood	Release Hypersensitivity
118	Cut-leaf Norway Maple (Emerald)	Release "Life Is Hard"
119	Maybush (Reeve's Spirea)	Female Self-Confidence
120	Maidenhair Tree	Release Inconsideration of Others

No.	Common Name	Primary Area of Essence Action
121	Weeping Maple	Lateral Thinking
122	White Horse Chestnut	Assists Kundalini
123	Weeping Mulberry	Unites Thought and Feeling
124	Spice Bush (Californian Allspice)	Obsessive Behaviors
125	Linden	Minor Substance Addiction
126	Oriental Liquidamber	Release Mental Reactivity
127	Burning Bush	Release Blame of Family
128	Korean Viburnum	Perception of Aging
129	Chinese Witch Hazel	Release "Busyness"
130	Turkistan Birch	Release Persistent Anxiety
131	Kentucky Coffee Tree	Acceptance of Body
132	Spiked Winter Hazel	Peer Group Pressure
133	Hornbeam	Release Superiority
134	Golden Elm	Lesser Obsessive Behaviors
135	Flowering Dogwood	Life Balance
136	Box Elder (Ghost Maple)	Value Emotions
137	Flowering Almond 'Double Crimson'	Dental Pain
138	African Laburnum	Skin Problems
139	David's Snake Bark Maple	Serious Viral Infections
140	Bleeding Heart Tree	Prostate
141	Silver Linden	Wound Healing
142	Indian Bean Tree	Foot Problems
143	Snowy Mespilus	Infertility
144	Snake Bark (Manchustriped Maple)	Blood Pressure
145	Silver Pear	Chronic Viral Infections
146	Weeping Mulberry	Varicose Veins
147	Holm Oak	Vascular Cleansing
148	Judas Tree	Lymphatic Cleansing
149	Valley Oak	Arm Problems
150	Scarlet Oak	Shoulder Problems
151	Liquidamber (Kallista)	Group Harmony
152	Chinese Wax Ash	Spiritual Connection
153	Horizontal Elm	Expanded Perspective
154	Photinia (Christmas Berry)	Focus
155	American Smoke Tree	Release Racism
156	Wheatley Elm (Jersey Elm)	Release Pain of Separation
157	Viburnum	Inner Confidence
158	Leatherwood	Patience
159	Autumn Zephyr-Lily (Flower of the West Wind)	Release Programmed Sexuality
160	Full Moon Maple	Emotional Awareness

TABLE 5.2: ALPHABETICAL LISTING OF COMMON NAMES OF TREES

No.	Common Name	Scientific Name
138	African Laburnum	*Calpurnia aurea*
74	American Nettle Tree (American Hackberry)	*Celtis occidentalis*
155	American Smoke Tree	*Cotinus obovatus*
14	Apricot	*Prunus armeniaca*
39	Aspen	*Populus tremula*
159	Autumn Zephyr-Lily (Flower of the West Wind)	*Zephyranthes candida*
79	Black Oak	*Quercus velutina*
23	Black Pussy Willow	*Salix x reichardtii* 'Nigra'
140	Bleeding Heart Tree	*Omalanthus populifolius*
136	Box Elder (Ghost Maple)	*Acer negundo*
73	Bradford Flowering Pear	*Pyrus calleryana* 'Bradford'
127	Burning Bush	*Euonymus alatus* 'Compactus'
111	Burr Oak (Mossy Cup Oak)	*Quercus macrocarpa*
50	Bush Cherry	*Prunus glandulosa*
60	Callery Pear	*Pyrus calleryana*
75	Camperdown Elm	*Ulmus glabra* 'Camperdownii'
112	Canoe Birch	*Betula papyrifera*
69	Celtic Cascade	*Salix x reichardtii* 'Pendula'
7	Cherry Plum	*Prunus cerasifera*
43	Chinese Elm	*Ulmus parvifolia*
76	Chinese Michelia	*Michelia doltsopa*
40	Chinese Trumpet Vine	*Campsis grandiflora*
152	Chinese Wax Ash	*Fraxinus chinensis*
129	Chinese Witch Hazel	*Hamamelis mollis*
1	Claret Ash	*Fraxinus angustifolia* 'Raywood'
84	Cockspur Hawthorn	*Crataegus crus-galli*
65	Common Hornbeam	*Carpinus betulus*
18	Copper Beech	*Fagus sylvatica* 'Purpurea'
53	Crab Apple	*Malus ioensis*
114	Crazy Filbert	*Corylus avellana* 'Contorta'
41	Crepe Myrtle	*Lagerstroemia indica*
106	Cut-leaf Birch	*Betula pendula* 'Dalecarlica'
118	Cut-leaf Norway Maple (Emerald)	*Acer platanoides* 'Lorbergii'
61	Cut-leaf Norway Maple (Sherbrooke)	*Acer platanoides* 'Lorbergii'
98	Cypress Oak	*Quercus robur* 'Fastigiata'
139	David's Snake Bark Maple	*Acer davidii*
48	Davy Filbert	*Corylus avelliana* 'Daviana'

No.	Common Name	Scientific Name
117	Dawn Redwood	*Metasequoia glyptostroboides*
15	Domestic Fig	*Ficus carica* 'White Adriatic'
3	Dove Tree	*Davidia involucrata*
56	Dutch Elm	*Ulmus x hollandica*
95	Eastern Red Bud	*Cercis canadensis*
25	Elderberry	*Sambuccus nigra*
11	English Elm	*Ulmus procera*
6	English Hawthorn	*Crataegus laevigata*
80	European Pussy Willow	*Salix discolor*
137	Flowering Almond 'Double Crimson'	*Prunus dulcis* 'Double Crimson'
82	Flowering Ash (Manna Ash)	*Fraxinus ornus*
90	Flowering Cherry	*Prunus serrulata* 'Mt Fuji'
135	Flowering Dogwood	*Cornus florida*
62	Flowering Peach	*Prunus persica* cv.
160	Full Moon Maple	*Acer japonicum*
22	Glory Vine	*Vitis coignetiae*
89	Golden Ash	*Fraxinus excelsior* 'Aurea'
134	Golden Elm	*Ulmus procera* 'Louis van Houtte'
116	Golden Italian Poplar	*Populus x canadensis* 'Serotina Aurea'
110	Golden Locust	*Robinia pseudoacacia* 'Frisia'
101	Green Honey Locust	*Gleditsia triacanthos* 'Shademaster'
91	Hedge Maple (Field Maple)	*Acer campestre*
147	Holm Oak	*Quercus ilex*
153	Horizontal Elm	*Ulmus glabra* 'Horizontalis'
133	Hornbeam	*Carpinus betulus* 'Fastigiata'
142	Indian Bean Tree	*Catalpa bignonioides*
83	Jacaranda	*Jacaranda acutifolia*
94	Japanese Barberry 'Golden Ring'	*Berberis thunbergii* 'Golden Ring'
33	Japanese Dogwood	*Cornus kousa*
81	Japanese Maple	*Acer palmatum*
87	Japanese Maple	*Acer palmatum* 'Omurayama'
36	Japanese White Birch	*Betula platyphylla* var. *japonica*
78	Japanese Zelkova	*Zelkova serrata*
148	Judas Tree	*Cercis siliquastrum*
131	Kentucky Coffee Tree	*Gymnocladus dioica*
96	Kilmarnock Willow	*Salix x reichardtii* 'Kilmarnock'
128	Korean Viburnum	*Viburnum carlesii*
158	Leatherwood	*Cyrilla racemiflora*
107	Lilac	*Syringa x hyacinthiflora*

No.	Common Name	Scientific Name
58	Lily-of-the-Valley Tree	*Clethra arborea*
46	Linden	*Tilia cordata* 'Greenspire'
125	Linden	*Tilia dasystyla*
2	Linden	*Tilia x europea*
10	Liquidamber (Donvale)	*Liquidambar styraciflua*
151	Liquidamber (Kallista)	*Liquidambar styraciflua*
21	Lombardy Poplar	*Populus nigra* var. *italica*
108	Magnolia 'Alexandrina'	*Magnolia x soulangeana* 'Alexandrina'
120	Maidenhair Tree	*Ginkgo biloba*
92	Manchurian Pear	*Pyrus ussuriensis*
119	Maybush (Reeve's Spirea)	*Spirea cantoniensis*
51	Mexican Hawthorn	*Crataegus pubescens*
126	Oriental Liquidamber	*Liquidambar orientalis*
16	Oriental Plane	*Platanus orientalis*
115	Pagoda Tree	*Sophora japonica* 'Pendula'
71	Peach	*Prunus persica*
27	Persian Witch Hazel (Persian Ironwood)	*Parrotia persica*
57	Persimmon	*Diospiros kaki*
154	Photinia (Christmas Berry)	*Photinia beauverdiana*
8	Pin Oak	*Quercus palustris*
13	Pink Horse Chestnut	*Aesculus x carnea*
34	Plane Tree	*Platanus racemosa*
59	Pomegranate	*Punica granatum*
45	Port Wine Magnolia	*Michelia figo*
104	Purple Leaf Pink Flowering Plum	*Prunus cerasifera* 'Nigra'
47	Purple Tulip Magnolia	*Magnolia liliflora* 'Nigra'
49	Purple Weeping Japanese Maple	*Acer palmatum* 'Dissectum Atropurpureum'
66	Pussy Willow (Goat Willow)	*Salix x reichardtii*
63	Red Cedar	*Toona ciliata*
38	Red Crepe Myrtle	*Lagerstroemia indica* 'Rubra'
42	Red Maple (Canadian Maple)	*Acer rubrum*
93	Red Oak	*Quercus rubra*
28	Rowan	*Sorbus aucuparia*
68	Sacred Yulan	*Magnolia denudata*
24	Sawtooth Oak (Bristle-tipped Oak)	*Quercus acutissima*
150	Scarlet Oak	*Quercus coccinea*
88	Scotch Elm	*Ulmus glabra*

No.	Common Name	Scientific Name
31	Silver Birch	*Betula pendula*
141	Silver Linden	*Tilia tomentosa*
32	Silver Maple	*Acer saccharinum*
145	Silver Pear	*Pyrus salicifolia*
55	Simon's Poplar	*Populus simonii* 'Fastigiata'
100	Smokebush	*Cotinus coggygria* 'Flame'
144	Snake Bark (Manchustriped Maple)	*Acer tegmentosum*
99	Snowball Tree (Guelder Rose)	*Viburnum opulus*
143	Snowy Mespilus	*Amelanchier canadensis*
97	Sorrell Tree (Sourwood)	*Oxydendrum arboreum*
124	Spice Bush (Californian Allspice)	*Calycanthus occidentalis*
132	Spiked Winter Hazel	*Corylopsis spicata*
86	Spring Cherry (Weeping Rosebud Cherry)	*Prunus pendula*
70	Star Magnolia	*Magnolia stellata*
54	Sugar Maple	*Acer saccharum*
37	Thornless Golden Honey Locust	*Gleditsia triacanthos* 'Sunburst'
35	Thornless Scarlet Honey Locust	*Gleditsia triacanthos* 'Ruby Lace'
77	Trident Maple	*Acer buergerianum*
26	Tulip Tree	*Liriodendron tulipifera*
67	Tupelo	*Nyssa sylvatica*
4	Turkey Oak	*Quercus cerris*
130	Turkistan Birch	*Betula turkistanica*
105	Ubame oak	*Quercus phillyraeoides*
149	Valley Oak	*Quercus lobata*
157	Viburnum	*Viburnum sieboldii*
44	Weeping Elm	*Ulmus glabra* 'Pendula'
17	Weeping Katsura Tree	*Cercidiphyllum japonicum* f. *pendulum*
121	Weeping Maple	*Acer palmatum* 'Red Filigree Lace'
102	Weeping Maple	*Acer palmatum* 'Sekimori'
146	Weeping Mulberry	*Morus alba* 'Pendula'
123	Weeping Mulberry	*Morus* sp.
5	Weeping Willow	*Salix babylonica*
156	Wheatley Elm (Jersey Elm)	*Ulmus minor* 'Sarniensis'
9	White Ash	*Fraxinus americana*
85	White Cedar	*Melia azedarach* var. *australasica*
109	White Flowering Dogwood	*Cornus florida* 'Alba'
72	White Flowering Plum	*Prunus cerasifera* 'Pissardii'
52	White Fringe Tree	*Chionanthus virginicus*
122	White Horse Chestnut	*Aesculus hippocastanum*

No.	Common Name	Scientific Name
30	White Mulberry	*Morus alba*
12	Willow Pattern Tree (Golden Rain Tree)	*Koelreuteria paniculata*
20	Winter Hazel	*Corylopsis sinensis* var. *calvescens*
113	Wintersweet (Allspice)	*Chimonanthus praecox*
64	Wisteria	*Wisteria sinensis*
29	Yeddo Cherry	*Prunus yedoensis*
19	Yellow Flowering Currant (Golden Currant)	*Ribes odoratum*
103	Young's Weeping Birch	*Betula pendula* 'Youngii'

TABLE 5.3: ALPHABETICAL LISTING OF SCIENTIFIC NAMES OF TREES

No.	Common Name	Scientific Name
77	Trident Maple	*Acer buergerianum*
91	Hedge Maple (Field Maple)	*Acer campestre*
139	David's Snake Bark Maple	*Acer davidii*
160	Full Moon Maple	*Acer japonicum*
136	Box Elder (Ghost Maple)	*Acer negundo*
81	Japanese Maple	*Acer palmatum*
49	Purple Weeping Japanese Maple	*Acer palmatum* 'Dissectum Atropurpureum'
87	Japanese Maple	*Acer palmatum* 'Omurayama'
121	Weeping Maple	*Acer palmatum* 'Red Filigree Lace'
102	Weeping Maple	*Acer palmatum* 'Sekimori'
61	Cut-leaf Norway Maple (Sherbrooke)	*Acer platanoides* 'Lorbergii'
118	Cut-leaf Norway Maple (Emerald)	*Acer platanoides* 'Lorbergii'
42	Red Maple (Canadian Maple)	*Acer rubrum*
32	Silver Maple	*Acer saccharinum*
54	Sugar Maple	*Acer saccharum*
144	Snake Bark (Manchustriped Maple)	*Acer tegmentosum*
122	White Horse Chestnut	*Aesculus hippocastanum*
13	Pink Horse Chestnut	*Aesculus x carnea*
143	Snowy Mespilus	*Amelanchier canadensis*
94	Japanese Barberry 'Golden Ring'	*Berberis thunbergii* 'Golden Ring'
130	Turkistan Birch	*Betula turkistanica*
112	Canoe Birch	*Betula papyrifera*
31	Silver Birch	*Betula pendula*
106	Cut-leaf Birch	*Betula pendula* 'Dalecarlica'
103	Young's Weeping Birch	*Betula pendula* 'Youngii'
36	Japanese White Birch	*Betula platyphylla* var. *japonica*
138	African Laburnum	*Calpurnia aurea*
124	Spice Bush (Californian Allspice)	*Calycanthus occidentalis*
40	Chinese Trumpet Vine	*Campsis grandiflora*
65	Common Hornbeam	*Carpinus betulus*
133	Hornbeam	*Carpinus betulus* 'Fastigiata'
142	Indian Bean Tree	*Catalpa bignonioides*
74	American Nettle Tree (American Hackberry)	*Celtis occidentalis*
17	Weeping Katsura Tree	*Cercidiphyllum japonicum* f. *pendulum*
95	Eastern Red Bud	*Cercis canadensis*
148	Judas Tree	*Cercis siliquastrum*
113	Wintersweet (Allspice)	*Chimonanthus praecox*
52	White Fringe Tree	*Chionanthus virginicus*

No.	Common Name	Scientific Name
58	Lily-of-the-Valley Tree	*Clethra arborea*
135	Flowering Dogwood	*Cornus florida*
109	White Flowering Dogwood	*Cornus florida* 'Alba'
33	Japanese Dogwood	*Cornus kousa*
20	Winter Hazel	*Corylopsis sinensis* var. *calvescens*
132	Spiked Winter Hazel	*Corylopsis spicata*
48	Davy Filbert	*Corylus avelliana* 'Daviana'
114	Crazy Filbert	*Corylus avellana* 'Contorta'
100	Smokebush	*Cotinus coggygria* 'Flame'
155	American Smoke Tree	*Cotinus obovatus*
84	Cockspur Hawthorn	*Crataegus crus-galli*
6	English Hawthorn	*Crataegus laevigata*
51	Mexican Hawthorn	*Crataegus pubescens*
158	Leatherwood	*Cyrilla racemiflora*
3	Dove Tree	*Davidia involucrata*
57	Persimmon	*Diospiros kaki*
127	Burning Bush	*Euonymus alatus* 'Compactus'
18	Copper Beech	*Fagus sylvatica* 'Purpurea'
15	Domestic Fig	*Ficus carica* 'White Adriatic'
9	White Ash	*Fraxinus americana*
1	Claret Ash	*Fraxinus angustifolia* 'Raywood'
152	Chinese Wax Ash	*Fraxinus chinensis*
89	Golden Ash	*Fraxinus excelsior* 'Aurea'
82	Flowering Ash (Manna Ash)	*Fraxinus ornus*
120	Maidenhair Tree	*Ginkgo biloba*
35	Thornless Scarlet Honey Locust	*Gleditsia triacanthos* 'Ruby Lace'
101	Green Honey Locust	*Gleditsia triacanthos* 'Shademaster'
37	Thornless Golden Honey Locust	*Gleditsia triacanthos* 'Sunburst'
131	Kentucky Coffee Tree	*Gymnocladus dioica*
129	Chinese Witch Hazel	*Hamamelis mollis*
83	Jacaranda	*Jacaranda acutifolia*
12	Willow Pattern Tree (Golden Rain Tree)	*Koelreuteria paniculata*
41	Crepe Myrtle	*Lagerstroemia indica*
38	Red Crepe Myrtle	*Lagerstroemia indica* 'Rubra'
126	Oriental Liquidamber	*Liquidambar orientalis*
10	Liquidamber (Donvale)	*Liquidambar styraciflua*
151	Liquidamber (Kallista)	*Liquidambar styraciflua*
26	Tulip Tree	*Liriodendron tulipifera*
68	Sacred Yulan	*Magnolia denudata*
47	Purple Tulip Magnolia	*Magnolia liliflora* 'Nigra'
70	Star Magnolia	*Magnolia stellata*
108	Magnolia 'Alexandrina'	*Magnolia* x *soulangeana* 'Alexandrina'

No.	Common Name	Scientific Name
53	Crab Apple	*Malus ioensis*
85	White Cedar	*Melia azedarach* var. *australasica*
117	Dawn Redwood	*Metasequoia glyptostroboides*
76	Chinese Michelia	*Michelia doltsopa*
45	Port Wine Magnolia	*Michelia figo*
30	White Mulberry	*Morus alba*
146	Weeping Mulberry	*Morus alba* 'Pendula'
123	Weeping Mulberry	*Morus* sp.
67	Tupelo	*Nyssa sylvatica*
140	Bleeding Heart Tree	*Omalanthus populifolius*
97	Sorrell Tree (Sourwood)	*Oxydendrum arboreum*
27	Persian Witch Hazel (Persian Ironwood)	*Parrotia persica*
154	Photinia (Christmas Berry)	*Photinia beauverdiana*
16	Oriental Plane	*Platanus orientalis*
34	Plane Tree	*Platanus racemosa*
21	Lombardy Poplar	*Populus nigra* var. *italica*
55	Simon's Poplar	*Populus simonii* 'Fastigiata'
39	Aspen	*Populus tremula*
116	Golden Italian Poplar	*Populus* x *canadensis* 'Serotina Aurea'
14	Apricot	*Prunus armeniaca*
7	Cherry Plum	*Prunus cerasifera*
104	Purple Leaf Pink Flowering Plum	*Prunus cerasifera* 'Nigra'
72	White Flowering Plum	*Prunus cerasifera* 'Pissardii'
137	Flowering Almond 'Double Crimson'	*Prunus dulcis* 'Double Crimson'
50	Bush Cherry	*Prunus glandulosa*
86	Spring Cherry (Weeping Rosebud Cherry)	*Prunus pendula*
71	Peach	*Prunus persica*
62	Flowering Peach	*Prunus persica* cv.
90	Flowering Cherry	*Prunus serrulata* 'Mt. Fuji'
29	Yeddo Cherry	*Prunus yedoensis*
59	Pomegranate	*Punica granatum*
60	Callery Pear	*Pyrus calleryana*
73	Bradford Flowering Pear	*Pyrus calleryana* 'Bradford'
145	Silver Pear	*Pyrus salicifolia*
92	Manchurian Pear	*Pyrus ussuriensis*
24	Sawtooth Oak (Bristle-tipped Oak)	*Quercus acutissima*
4	Turkey Oak	*Quercus cerris*
150	Scarlet Oak	*Quercus coccinea*
147	Holm Oak	*Quercus ilex*
149	Valley Oak	*Quercus lobata*

No.	Common Name	Scientific Name
111	Burr Oak (Mossy Cup Oak)	*Quercus macrocarpa*
8	Pin Oak	*Quercus palustris*
105	Ubame oak	*Quercus phillyraeoides*
98	Cypress Oak	*Quercus robur* 'Fastigiata'
93	Red Oak	*Quercus rubra*
79	Black Oak	*Quercus velutina*
19	Yellow Flowering Currant (Golden Currant)	*Ribes odoratum*
110	Golden Locust	*Robinia pseudoacacia* 'Frisia'
5	Weeping Willow	*Salix babylonica*
80	European Pussy Willow	*Salix discolor*
66	Pussy Willow (Goat Willow)	*Salix x reichardtii*
96	Kilmarnock Willow	*Salix x reichardtii* 'Kilmarnock'
23	Black Pussy Willow	*Salix x reichardtii* 'Nigra'
69	Celtic Cascade	*Salix x reichardtii* 'Pendula'
25	Elderberry	*Sambuccus nigra*
115	Pagoda Tree	*Sophora japonica* 'Pendula'
28	Rowan	*Sorbus aucuparia*
119	Maybush (Reeve's Spirea)	*Spirea cantoniensis*
107	Lilac	*Syringa x hyacinthiflora*
46	Linden	*Tilia cordata* 'Greenspire'
125	Linden	*Tilia dasystyla*
141	Silver Linden	*Tilia tomentosa*
2	Linden	*Tilia x europea*
63	Red Cedar	*Toona ciliata*
88	Scotch Elm	*Ulmus glabra*
75	Camperdown Elm	*Ulmus glabra* 'Camperdownii'
153	Horizontal Elm	*Ulmus glabra* 'Horizontalis'
44	Weeping Elm	*Ulmus glabra* 'Pendula'
156	Wheatley Elm (Jersey Elm)	*Ulmus minor* 'Sarniensis'
43	Chinese Elm	*Ulmus parvifolia*
11	English Elm	*Ulmus procera*
134	Golden Elm	*Ulmus procera* 'Louis van Houtte'
56	Dutch Elm	*Ulmus x hollandica*
128	Korean Viburnum	*Viburnum carlesii*
99	Snowball Tree (Guelder Rose)	*Viburnum opulus*
157	Viburnum	*Viburnum sieboldii*
22	Glory Vine	*Vitis coignetiae*
64	Wisteria	*Wisteria sinensis*
78	Japanese Zelkova	*Zelkova serrata*
159	Autumn Zephyr-Lily (Flower of the West Wind)	*Zephyranthes candida*

TABLE 5.4: EMOTIONS AND CORRESPONDING FALLING LEAF ESSENCES

Released Emotion	FLE No.	Common Name
Anger	14	Apricot
Anxiety	77	Trident Maple
Bitterness	93	Red Oak
Dependency	113	Wintersweet
Depression	80	European Pussy Willow
Detachment	107	Lilac
Disappointment	35	Thornless Scarlet Honey Locust
Dislike	114	Crazy Filbert
Disillusion	91	Hedge Maple
Emotional Awareness	160	Full Moon Maple
Emotional Turmoil	44	Weeping Elm
Envy	36	Japanese White Birch
Fear of Abandonment	95	Eastern Red Bud
Fear of Aging	108	Magnolia 'Alexandrina'
Fear of Change	16	Oriental Plane
Fear of Commitment	104	Purple Leaf Pink Flowering Plum
Fear of Dependency	96	Kilmarnock Willow
Fear of Disability	100	Smokebush
Fear of Disappointment	105	Ubame Oak
Fear of Dying	98	Cypress Oak
Fear of Happiness	103	Young's Weeping Birch
Fear of Illness	99	Snowball Tree
Fear of Imperfection	97	Sorrell Tree
Fear of Inadequacy	111	Burr Oak
Fear of Lack of Love	42	Red Maple
Fear of Loneliness	110	Golden Locust
Fear of Losing Face	109	White Flowering Dogwood
Fear of Loss	106	Cut-leaf Birch
Fear of Love	17	Weeping Katsura Tree
Fear of Poverty	94	Japanese Barberry 'Golden Ring'
Fear of Rejection	101	Green Honey Locust
Fear of the Unknown	40	Chinese Trumpet Vine
Grief	92	Manchurian Pear
Guilt	15	Domestic Fig
Hatred	18	Copper Beech
Inadequacy	102	Weeping Maple
Intolerance	116	Golden Italian Poplar
Jealousy	37	Thornless Golden Honey Locust
Loneliness	39	Aspen

Released Emotion	FLE No.	Common Name
Pain of Separation	156	Wheatley Elm
Persistent Anxiety	130	Turkistan Birch
Possessiveness	38	Red Crepe Myrtle
Revenge	115	Pagoda Tree
Sadness	73	Bradford Flowering Pear
Uncertainty	41	Crepe Myrtle

TABLE 5.5: PHYSICAL IMBALANCES AND CORRESPONDING FALLING LEAF ESSENCES

Physical Imbalance	FLE No.	Common Name
After Stroke	59	Pomegranate
After Surgery	28	Rowan
Arm Problems	149	Valley Oak
Arteries/Veins	55	Simon's Poplar
Back	66	Pussy Willow (Goat Willow)
Bladder Incontinence	78	Japanese Zelkova
Blood Pressure	144	Snake Bark
Breasts	32	Silver Maple
Cellulite	86	Spring Cherry
Chest	52	White Fringe Tree
Chronic Viral Infections	145	Silver Pear
Conjunctivitis	79	Black Oak
Dental Pain	137	Flowering Almond 'Double Crimson'
Emphysema/Recurrent Chest Infection	81	Japanese Maple
Endocrine System	4	Turkey Oak
Eyes—Deterioration	82	Flowering Ash (Manna Ash)
Fatigue	7	Cherry Plum
Female Reproductive System	11	English Elm
Fluid Retention	13	Pink Horse Chestnut
Foot Problems	142	Indian Bean Tree
Gout	33	Japanese Dogwood
Hair Loss	85	White Cedar
Headache	67	Tupelo
Heart	26	Tulip Tree
Indigestion	34	Plane Tree
Infertility	143	Snowy Mespilus
Inflammation	10	Liquidamber (Donvale)
Influenza	1	Claret Ash

Physical Imbalance	FLE No.	Common Name
Injury	63	Red Cedar
Insomnia	68	Sacred Yulan
Irritable Bowel	87	Japanese Maple
Kidneys	5	Weeping Willow
Large Intestine	65	Common Hornbeam
Liver	64	Wisteria
Lymphatic Cleansing	148	Judas Tree
Malignancy	58	Lily-of-the-Valley Tree
Muscular Weakness	30	White Mulberry
Nausea	69	Celtic Cascade
Nervous Insomnia	12	Willow Pattern Tree
Osteoarthritis	9	White Ash
Osteoporosis	75	Camperdown Elm
Pancreas	76	Chinese Michelia
Prostate (More Serious Problems)	62	Flowering Peach
Prostate	140	Bleeding Heart Tree
Rheumatoid Arthritis	70	Star Magnolia
Serious Viral Infection	139	David's Snake Bark Maple
Shoulder Problems	150	Scarlet Oak
Sinuses	74	American Nettle Tree
Skin Problems	138	African Laburnum
Skin, Ears, Nose, Throat	61	Cut-leaf Norway Maple (Sherbrooke)
Snoring	84	Cockspur Hawthorn
Substance Addiction	21	Lombardy Poplar
Substance Addiction (Minor)	125	Linden *(Tilia dasystyla)*
Tonic	2	Linden *(Tilia x europea)*
Tumors	50	Bush Cherry
Varicose Veins	146	Weeping Mulberry
Vascular Cleansing	147	Holm Oak
Veins/Capillaries	54	Sugar Maple
Wounds	141	Silver Linden

6 Complex and Combination Falling Leaf Essences

SOME ESSENCE PRESCRIBERS WILL THRIVE on the detail presented in the previous chapter. Indeed, an enthusiastic essence practitioner can easily assemble five hundred to two thousand essences of different types. Others will throw up their hands in despair at the notion of a list of 160 falling leaf essences from which they must select. For better or for worse, the world in which we live moves faster and faster. The clamor is not for greater detail and complexity, but rather for something that can be decided simply from a limited range of options. It is to meet this need for simplicity that I have developed the following range of thirty-eight combination and complex essences. They have been developed around the most recurrent themes of need that I see as an essence practitioner. One can then choose whether to work using individual falling leaf essences, or to use the combinations below, or to use both (at different times). These formulations are proprietary to my company Advanced Alchemy Pty. Ltd., but I share the information knowing that readers will use it in ways that are appropriate.

The essences described in this chapter fall into two basic types: combination essences and complex essences. These are available in dosage strength, that is, an essence that is ready to be taken and does not require dilution.

Combination essences are combinations of falling leaf essences; they are sometimes also combined with bark essences, seed essences, and snow-modified Australian flower essences. The concept is simple in principle but somewhat more demanding in practice. For example, it is an art to produce a combination essence that has the required stability to last at least a year or two in its shelf life. All combinations are sufficiently stable to ingest right away, but many begin to deteriorate after one to nine months if they are not made appropriately.

Complex essences are those essences that are generated in a number of sequential steps. For example, we could say that flower essences belong to the simple essences. There is basically just one step to the process—the flowers are placed in water in the sunlight. Falling leaf essences also belong to the simple essences, as here, too, there is basically just one step to the process. The snow-modified Australian flower essences, by contrast, are two-step essences. In the first step, a classical flower essence is made. In the second, that essence is modified by placing it in the snow for several hours. As we have seen, this generates an essence very different from the original flower essence. Essences that are made in two or more sequential steps I refer to as complex essences. Those made in a single step are simple essences. It does not necessarily follow that complex essences are better than simple essences; again, it depends on the nature of the task in hand.

However, the notion of complex essences is a very exciting one. It means that one can, as it were, tailor-make an essence for a particular purpose by permutating preexisting nature energies in a defined sequence. Sometimes the sequence of steps acts like a step-up transformer in an electrical system. At other times the sequence of steps enables one to generate an essence capable of working in different ways on different levels around the problem in hand. In making complex essences, we are looking at the water molecule as a programmable medium for storing coded instructions that the body then reads and enacts by following the requested changes. An analogy helpful to understanding the difference between simple and complex essences is to consider a simple flower essence or falling leaf essence as one note on the piano. A complex essence is more like a sequence of notes or a concerto. As in composing music for the piano, there are certain principles, but ultimately one must have a "feel" for musical composition. So it is with complex essences: The process of invention has certain aspects of science and particularly chemistry, but ultimately one must have a "feel" for the flow of steps required.

Please note that there are several essences in the listing below that are just simple essences. These are entitled "Protection from Electromagnetic Radiation," "Coping with the News," and "Conflicts at Work," each of which is represented by a single, simple bark essence. The reason for their inclusion is that these are important topics, and these simple essences are in my opinion fully adequate to meet these needs. Combination and complex essences can be excellent, but when a simple essence will do the job, use it!

The recommended adult dosage for combination and complex essences is generally 7 drops under the tongue three times daily.

Please note that all these essences are trademark and copyright protected.

Abundance and Ease

The consciousness of abundance and an ease with life are encouraged by this combination of falling leaf essences.

CONSTITUENT ESSENCES

Falling Leaf Essences

#31 Silver Birch	Release struggle
#94 Japanese Barberry 'Golden Ring'	Release fear of poverty

Anti-*Candida*

This complex essence works effectively in combination with appropriate dietary measures to balance the overgrowth of *Candida* yeast cells in the body.

Arthritis Formula

Arthritis Formula is a combination of snow-modified Australian flower essences that can be used for the relief of the aches and pains of both osteo- and rheumatoid arthritis.

CONSTITUENT ESSENCES

Snow-Modified Australian Flower Essences

Small-leaf Guinea Flower	Bones
Native Violet	Heart
Sidney Rock Rose	Immune system
Blue Lechenanlita	Muscles

Becoming Your Own Person

This combination of falling leaf essences facilitates the process of individuation, or moving away from how you have been programmed, by family and society, to become who you really are.

CONSTITUENT ESSENCES

Falling Leaf Essences

#20 Winter Hazel	Release programmed living
#29 Yeddo Cherry	Mental flexibility
#127 Burning Bush	Release blame of family
#132 Spiked Winter Hazel	Peer group pressure

Cassandra's Apple

The base of this complex essence is the Bach flower remedy Crab Apple. Cassandra's Apple assists with hormonal balance, menopause, premenstrual tension, and other menstrual cycle–related symptoms.

Cellular Regeneration

This complex essence is used to rebuild and renew tissues, especially after stress and change. It also imparts energy and stamina.

Chronic Fatigue

This combination of falling leaf essences is designed to help in chronic fatigue syndrome. It can also help those who feel plain worn out.

CONSTITUENT ESSENCES

Falling Leaf Essences

#2 Linden	Tonic
#4 Turkey Oak	Endocrine System
#5 Weeping Willow	Kidneys
#8 Pin Oak	Fatigue
#26 Tulip Tree	Heart
#30 White Mulberry	Muscular weakness

Conflicts at Work

This bark essence (Liquidamber) protects one in the workplace from politics and conflicts both seen and unseen. It keeps one from being inappropriately drawn into such situations because of emotional attachments.

Coping with the News

The bark essence of Pin Oak lends protection from the constant bombardment of information we face every day on the overwhelming political, social, and environmental issues on both the national and international fronts.

Emotional Well-being

This combination of falling leaf essences nurtures the emotional level to generate a profound sense of well-being.

CONSTITUENT ESSENCES

Falling Leaf Essences

#2 Linden	Tonic
#7 Cherry Plum	Emotional well-being
#44 Weeping Elm	Release emotional turmoil
#126 Oriental Liquidamber	Release mental reactivity

Emma's Rose

Emma's Rose is a complex essence used to help one rebuild from long-term stress, nervous depletion, and emotional exhaustion. It is based on the gem hematite and the Alaskan flower essence Bog Rosemary.

Explovir

This complex essence targets active viruses in the human system. It can be used to treat colds, the flu, herpes, shingles, and other persistent viral infections.

Fear of the Unknown

When one is faced with huge change or is forced to let go of the familiar without having anything to replace it, fear of the unknown arises. This combination of falling leaf essences helps with the terror of stepping off the cliff and entering free fall.

CONSTITUENT ESSENCES

Falling Leaf Essences

#16 Oriental Plane	Release fear of change
#40 Chinese Trumpet Vine	Release fear of the unknown
#98 Cypress Oak	Release fear of dying
#106 Cut-leaf Birch	Release fear of loss

Finding New Directions

At a loss as to what to do next or where the road leads from here? This combination of seed essences will help new things germinate in your life; over time, new directions will emerge.

CONSTITUENT ESSENCES

Seed Essences

Turkey Oak	Releases hidden potential
English Elm	Assists in refining creative pathway
Weeping Katsura Tree	Releases blocks in creativity
Chinese Trumpet Vine	Opens one up to a new level of creativity
Davy Filbert	Opens one up to the expression of spirit

Grounding Essence

This is an important complex essence for today's stressful lifestyle. It can assist us in dealing with the many stressful situations that cause us to become ungrounded and unable to think and act clearly.

Help for Addictions

Wherever you lie on the scale of addiction, from the delights of chocolate, tea, and coffee to something stronger, this combination of falling leaf essences help balance the addictive tendency. It is also very useful for addictive or compulsive behaviors.

CONSTITUENT ESSENCES

Falling Leaf Essences

#21 Lombardy Poplar	Substance addiction
#124 Spice Bush	Obsessive behaviors
#125 Linden	Minor substance addiction
#134 Golden Elm	Lesser obsessive behaviors

Help for Anxiety/Panic Attacks

This combination of falling leaf essences, snow-modified Australian flower essences, and a bark essence assists when a person is experiencing an anxiety or panic attack. It helps calm and neutralize the overwhelming emotions. Take 7 drops every five to ten minutes in an acute situation.

CONSTITUENT ESSENCES

Falling Leaf Essences

#16 Oriental Plane	Release fear of change
#77 Trident Maple	Anxiety
#130 Turkistan Birch	Release Persistent anxiety

Snow-Modified Australian Flower Essences

Native Violet	Heart
Fringed Heath Myrtle	Central nervous system

Bark Essence

White Ash	Helps one to see that there are choices

Help for Depression

This combination essence can help ease the "blues," states of despondency, and possibly discouragement. It consists of two falling leaf essences and two snow-modified Australian flower essences.

CONSTITUENT ESSENCES

Falling Leaf Essences

#7 Cherry Plum	Emotional well-being
#80 European Pussy Willow	Depression

Snow-Modified Australian Flower Essences

Native Violet	Heart
Fringed Heath Myrtle	Central nervous system

Ice Calcite Essence

Ice Calcite is used to treat persistent, longstanding health problems. It is particularly helpful in treating conditions that seem resistant to other therapy. It produces the "big thaw" for a frozen state.

Improve Study

To help fulfill one's potential in mastering new information, this combination of falling leaf essences seeks to keep the brain active, alert, and focused.

CONSTITUENT ESSENCES

Falling Leaf Essences

#29 Yeddo Cherry	Mental flexibility
#56 Dutch Elm	Mental functions
#121 Weeping Maple	Lateral thinking
#154 Photinia	Focus
#158 Leatherwood	Patience

Injuries/Wounds

Try this combination of falling leaf essences to ease the pain of strains and sprains, bruising, and bad backs and to help the healing of cuts and wounds.

CONSTITUENT ESSENCES

Falling Leaf Essences

#10 Liquidamber	Inflammation
#63 Red Cedar	Injury
#66 Pussy Willow	Back
#141 Silver Linden	Wound healing

Interpersonal Harmony Essence

This complex essence helps purify or cleanse the energy between two people. Only one person needs to take the essence, although both can, if appropriate.

Loss and Grief

This combination of falling leaf essences is recommended for bereavement and for other losses that occur in life, including loss of a relationship, loss of employment, and loss of a pet. It helps with adjustment and the stages of the grieving process.

CONSTITUENT ESSENCES

Falling Leaf Essences

#3 Dove Tree	Bereavement
#26 Tulip Tree	Heart
#51 Mexican Hawthorn	Death
#92 Manchurian Pear	Release grief

OBA Elixir

This complex essence is based on the gems obsidian (O), bloodstone (B), and amber (A). It is suitable for short- and long-term usage for building energy and stamina.

Pain Relief Complex

This complex essence can be used to ease short-term discomfort. It excels in long-term pain relief in chronic cases—just keep taking it.

Personal Growth

A gentle encouragement to personal growth, reflection, life balance, and spirituality is afforded by this combination of falling leaf essences.

CONSTITUENT ESSENCES

Falling Leaf Essences

#31 Silver Birch	Release struggle
#47 Purple Tulip Magnolia	Spirituality
#71 Peach	Personal growth
#90 Flowering Cherry	Reflection
#135 Flowering Dogwood	Life balance

Physical Detoxification

In this era of environmental pollution, it is helpful periodically to detoxify the physical body. This combination of falling leaf essences brings about a release of toxins from major body organs and tissues.

CONSTITUENT ESSENCES

Falling Leaf Essences

#5 Weeping Willow	Kidneys
#26 Tulip Tree	Heart
#64 Wisteria	Liver
#147 Holm Oak	Vascular cleansing
#148 Judas Tree	Lymphatic cleansing

Preserving Self-Esteem

This combination of the bark essences Canadian Maple and Turkey Oak affords protection from fierce attacks on self-esteem. It filters out the projection of failure from people who seek to undermine a person and his or her self-esteem. It is especially useful in cases where others seek to keep a person within an expected mold.

Protection from Electromagnetic Radiation

The remarkable bark essence of Scarlet Oak protects one against electronic radiation from computers and many other everyday technologies, electromagnetic ley lines, other earth energies, and also subliminal programming.

Release Anger

This combination of falling leaf essences helps the volatile or inflammatory emotions including anger to be mobilized and released. Physical exercise and verbal expression of feelings can help these emotions to dissipate. Sometimes a bath or a shower can be helpful. Generally speaking, as with all falling leaf essences, the extent of the response is proportional to dosage. Therefore, reduce the dosage or stop taking the essence for a few days if the volatile emotions are too strong.

CONSTITUENT ESSENCES

Falling Leaf Essences

#14 Apricot	Release anger
#37 Thornless Golden Honey Locust	Release jealousy
#64 Wisteria	Liver
#93 Red Oak	Release bitterness
#115 Pagoda Tree	Release revenge

Release Control

This falling leaf essence combination helps those who suffer from the stress of needing to control the events, circumstances, and people in their lives.

CONSTITUENT ESSENCES

Falling Leaf Essences

#22 Glory Vine	Release mental control
#38 Red Crepe Myrtle	Release possessiveness
#49 Purple Weeping Japanese Maple	Perfectionism

Release Guilt

Guilt can be a difficult and immobilizing emotion arising from old conditioning. This combination of two falling leaf essences facilitates the release of guilt from both the mind and the body.

CONSTITUENT ESSENCES

Falling Leaf Essences

#15 Domestic Fig	Release guilt
#26 Tulip Tree	Heart

Respiratory Essence

This complex essence can be used to treat respiratory disorders, including asthma, croup, influenza, hay fever, and rhinitis.

Self-Esteem

A strong self-esteem is necessary for success and happiness in life. This combination of falling leaf essences builds self-esteem and aids in the release of past issues that have had an adverse effect.

CONSTITUENT ESSENCES

Falling Leaf Essences

#19 Yellow Flowering Currant	Self-esteem
#23 Black Pussy Willow	Specific low self-esteem
#48 Davy Filbert	Physical self-image
#102 Weeping Maple	Release inadequacy
#119 Maybush	Female self-confidence
#133 Hornbeam	Release superiority

Sexuality

This combination of falling leaf essences works to improve self-image and acceptance of the body, ease with sexuality, and libido. It also aids the release of inappropriate conditioning or programming in the area of sexuality.

CONSTITUENT ESSENCES

Falling Leaf Essences

#25 Elderberry	Sexuality
#46 Linden	Release chauvinism
#48 Davy Filbert	Physical self-image
#83 Jacaranda	Sex drive
#131 Kentucky Coffee Tree	Acceptance of body
#159 Autumn Zephyr-Lily	Release programmed sexuality

Shock and Trauma Remedy

When an emergency, shock, or trauma is experienced, this combination of falling leaf, snow-modified Australian flower, and bark essences can act as a buffer to both the shock and the trauma. It assists realignment and rebalancing. Seven drops can be taken every five to ten minutes when in acute need.

CONSTITUENT ESSENCES

Falling Leaf Essences

#7 Cherry Plum	Emotional well-being
#40 Chinese Trumpet Vine	Release fear of the unknown

Snow-Modified Australian Flower Essences

Epacris reclinata	Adrenals
Native Violet	Heart
Fringed Heath Myrtle	Central nervous system

Bark Essence

Pin Oak	Assists with the filtering of external stresses

Skin Problems

This combination of falling leaf essences helps with skin problems, including eczema, dermatitis, rashes, skin bumps and blemishes, and psoriasis. Its actions are directed partly toward the skin and partly to the systems that support it, such as the liver and lymphatic systems.

CONSTITUENT ESSENCES

Falling Leaf Essences

#10 Liquidamber	Inflammation
#64 Wisteria	Liver
#138 African Laburnum	Skin problems
#148 Judas Tree	Lymphatic cleansing

Transcendence

This complex essence is designed to encourage detachment in difficult or stressful life circumstances. It is very helpful for those who suffer from emotional overinvolvement.

7

Making and Storing
Falling Leaf Essences

MAKING FALLING LEAF ESSENCES is not at all difficult. In the space of a day or two, a high school science student could be taught how to do it competently. The processes are not far removed from common procedures of chemistry and botany classrooms. But there is far more involved in making falling leaf essences than simple chemistry and botany. It requires an appropriate consciousness and attitude. Even more important, it requires relationship with the plants. Paradoxically, the greater the scientific training one has had, the more difficult the process becomes, because it becomes difficult to accept a basic tenet: Making falling leaf essences is 10 percent chemistry and 90 percent relationship.

The Psychic Energy of Trees

Most people believe that plants have little consciousness or awareness. People who talk to plants are generally looked upon as being rather odd. Even more peculiar are people who claim that plants talk back to them! Obviously, plants have no mouth to speak with in order to get our attention. If plants do have consciousness and do seek to communicate, they must do so on a more subtle, invisible level, rather like telepathy. Clearly, if one believes or has been programmed to believe that plants are nonintelligent life-forms without significant consciousness, one will unknowingly obstruct such subtle communication from the outset.

In my initial attempts to make falling leaf essences, I approached the project as if it were simply a matter of chemistry and botany. I soon came to regret the error of my ways, because the energies I experienced during the process were decidedly unpleasant. A scientist should be aware of both the visible aspects of his work and the subtle energies around it. If necessary, new hypotheses must be considered and implemented in response to this realm of subtle energy.

One who is sensitive to the more subtle levels of energy will be well aware of the ability of plants, particularly trees, to generate hostile energy or even psychic attack upon those who seek to destroy or harm them. It is as though trees, quite helpless to defend themselves against a major aggressor in the physical realm, have, through the processes of evolution, become quite expert in organizing and using subtle, invisible psychic energies as a web of protection. Having repeatedly experienced these subtle energies, I suggest that the tree is at least able to sense or interpret whether a person or animal poses a threat.

In the esoteric view of plants, quite a complex understanding has been developed around nature spirits that work with and through the plant kingdom. These spirits, sometimes called devas, are considered to be invisible, conscious, intelligent sentient beings. Devas could be the source of some of the psychic energy that trees use as protection.

Of course the notion of trees possessing such a refined, defensive consciousness is far removed from the collective mind-set of most botanists and scientists. However, in essence work, one is not unduly swayed by popular scientific opinion. Indeed, one would not do the research work at all if one were encumbered by scientific opinion— there is no paradigm in science at present to support or explain the very existence of essences!

If one begins to make falling leaf essences as if this were simply an exercise in chemistry, the energies around the preparation process become increasingly difficult. The energetic intensity can actually make one become physically ill. It is as though seeking to extract a tree's spirit or life force without properly tuning in to its energy activates that tree's psychic defense mechanisms. Sometimes this energetic intensity occurs as the leaves are placed in water. On other occasions it occurs as one approaches a tree with merely a possible intention of gathering its falling leaves. It can even occur a day or two before one has located a particular tree.

Four relevant hypotheses about trees' energetic reaction can be made. First, people who are less attuned to the subtle levels of energy will probably be less affected by them in an adverse way. Second, this energetic reaction may be maximal when one is trying something new. For example, flower essences have been made hundreds and even thousands of times, and now it is a process that occurs easily and without resistance. It is as though the flowering plants have grown accustomed to this process and more or less given it the nod of acceptance. But when Edward Bach first tuned in to the appropriate plants, he went through extremes of mental, emotional, and physical suffering. Through this suffering, the nature of the essence of each flower was revealed. Yet one could equally understand this experience as a psychic attack from the essence or deva of that particular plant, resisting tooth and nail the coming extraction of its essence for human use. Falling leaf essences are a relatively new creation; they have not been prepared on a widespread, ongoing basis. It is as though the trees react out of a primal fear of something fundamentally new or different being done with their energy. The situation is rather analogous to being given the task of riding a stallion that has never been broken in. Initially the ride is very rough, but subsequent riders have a much easier time. Through the process of being broken in, the horse overcomes its extreme fear and panic.

Third, one can hypothesize on the basis of experience that this energetic reaction or psychic attack from the tree can be minimized or avoided altogether by relating to the tree on an ongoing basis on the subtle, telepathic level. The subtle level of telepathic interaction with trees reveals a consciousness that is profoundly skeptical of the intention of human beings. Of course, the trees have suffered centuries of use and abuse by humans without any consultation with the trees themselves or with the nature spirits. They may perceive humans as acting without consideration of their interests. When one actually approaches a tree with a desire to interact telepathically, the first feeling

Falling leaf essences are most commonly prepared from the fallen leaves of deciduous trees. However, the distinction between "evergreen" and "deciduous" is not clear-cut. Some deciduous trees do not lose all their leaves, while some true evergreens lose some leaves in certain seasons as part of their growth and replacement program. What matters is not the category but the energy of the leaf; it falls for a reason, and that reason generates the energy that imbues the falling leaf essence. Therefore, falling leaf essences can also be prepared from evergreen trees and shrubs at certain times.

one receives in response is sometimes that of genuine surprise. It is as if the tree is thinking, "What, a human being who respects and wants to talk with me?"

Fourth, the strength of the psychic reaction appears to be proportional to the number of essences being made simultaneously. At some points, I and my colleagues undertook to make ten to fifteen essences simultaneously. This is not to be recommended! The psychic force that many trees together can muster is truly formidable and possibly engages the collective consciousness of other related groups of trees. It is better to make just one, two, or, at the most, three essences at a time. In terms of maintaining conscious telepathic relationship with the trees from which essences are being extracted, this is a much more manageable number.

Establishing Relationship with Trees

The process of establishing dialogue with trees from which one wants to extract an essence is very similar to seeking cooperation in a venture from other human beings. One has to show them and explain to them that this venture will benefit them, too. They need to be shown the positive aspect of the outcome and, if they have fears, be patiently reassured. The benefits of entering this quiet process of negotiation and counseling with the trees are immense. When one proceeds to make essences with the cooperation of the trees, it is a gentle and enjoyable experience. On the contrary, if one proceeds arrogantly to make the essences without consulting the trees, the essences are made in an environment of conflict, misunderstanding, and hostility—which must have some effect on the quality and nature of the resulting essence.

To those who are skeptical of the idea of communicating with plants, it can only be said that they need to experience the process for themselves. Like enlightenment, communication with the plant kingdom and the consequences of doing so, or not doing so, must ultimately be experienced to be understood.

Selecting a Tree

The selection of an appropriate tree for essence collection can occur in one of two ways. Sometimes one goes out having decided upon the destination and having decided in advance to collect falling leaves. On other occasions, one observes a tree while out for another purpose and feels it appropriate to collect falling leaves from that tree at that time or later. I have found trees suitable for falling leaf collection at a number of locations: the Royal Botanical Gardens in Melbourne, the Dandenongs (a very beautiful and heavily treed area in the outer suburbs of Melbourne), Bright, private gardens in and around Melbourne, and advanced tree nurseries.

There exist purists who believe that the tree or plant used for essence collection should be found far from any human habitation or industry. This hypothetical tree exists in pristine splendor, free of exposure to soil, water, and air pollution. But requiring such a purity of environment is totally unrealistic when it comes to falling leaf essence collection. The overwhelming percentage of trees suitable for falling leaf collection are deciduous trees whose origins lie in the Northern Hemisphere. Those that I have used in Australia were transplanted to this continent and placed quite deliberately in and around human habitation to be admired by people. They do not exist in remote and pristine splendor in the untouched heart of the Australian Bush. On the contrary, because these deciduous trees of Northern

Hemisphere origin exist around human habitation, they are somewhat adapted to humanity, and using essences from them is a further step in a process of interrelationship with humans initiated long ago.

One must simply be sensible when collecting falling leaf essences. Trees located near busy roadways or freeways, factories, and obvious sources of local pollution should be avoided. Other than these, a strong case can be made that the most effective plants for essence preparation are those found living near human habitation. Some herbalists believe that the plants growing quite spontaneously in your backyard, or in a vacant lot down the street, are in fact exactly what you need. Some plants may be needed on an herbal (physical) level, others on an energetic (essence) level. In this view, there exists some spontaneous law of attraction between humans and the plants that they need for well-being. While accepting this argument in its general sense, I certainly don't suggest that you take it literally to the extent of preparing an herbal cocktail from all the weeds in that vacant lot down the street!

Storing Essences

After an essence has been extracted in water, that water is combined with ethanol (becoming the "falling leaf essence stock"), stored in wine bottles, and corked until use. We store these wine bottles on wooden modular racks, like those used in the wine industry, in a specially designed room. The room and floor are made out of cedar and untreated pine, because the stocks last longer in environments that have plenty of wood. There is no permanent electricity supply to the room, and plastic and synthetic substances are avoided wherever possible. The temperature in the room is not allowed to rise beyond 30 degrees Centigrade. This is a cautionary measure, as the stocks appear to be temperature tolerant up to at least 35 degrees Centigrade. It is likely that falling leaf essence stocks will last for ten to twenty years under such suitable conditions.

The essence stocks, like the trees from which they were extracted, have their own consciousness. Indeed, the essences could be regarded as noncellular life-forms. When visiting the room filled with falling leaf essence stocks, one is impressed by the power of this collective consciousness. There seems to be a very clear communication from the essence stocks when they are not happy with some aspect of their environment. For the first six months following their creation, essence stocks appear to be somewhat volatile and unpredictable in their consciousness; after that, they "settle down." For this reason, we prefer to keep new essence stocks in the room for about six months before dispensing them in smaller bottles to clients. Over this time, a relationship of trust is formed between human and essence. Each time one enters this essence room, one is aware of one's relationship with the essences stored there.

Making Falling Leaf Essences

Three people have been intensely involved in making falling leaf essences: myself, Trudi Dempsey, and Jennie Richardson. In the following section, Jennie gives her perspectives on the making of falling leaf essences.

"In Memory of All Trees"

by Jennie Richardson

It is with great respect that I write of my experiences about the making of the falling leaf essences. I wish to honor the energies that I work with to create these essences: the tree devas, the nature spirits, and the elements of air, earth, water, and fire. Without a harmony and cooperation with these energies, the falling leaf essences would not have been created.

We must do much groundwork, building our relationship with the devas and elementals, before we go out to find the appropriate trees that are ready in their autumn splendor. Just as there is a code of behavior and ethics we must adhere to when entering a foreign culture, so too is there a code of behavior and ethics we must learn before entering the realm of nature. We cannot just bowl into another culture and do what we like without regard for that culture's customs; so, too, we cannot successfully attune and harmonize with the nature realm unless we observe and follow its protocols.

It should be noted that essences occur naturally, and not only as a consequence of essence-making activities by humans. For example, if one finds a pond, lake, or stream in a forested environment in autumn, one may well find a number of leaves from deciduous trees floating on its surface. This is all that is required for the stream or lake water to be imbued with several falling leaf essences. Plant and fish life in the stream, along with birds and animals that drink from this body of water, will ingest these falling leaf essences. The dew that falls from the flowering parts of plants contains a flower essence. Bodies and even droplets of water with a sufficient presence of seeds will contain seed essences.

The realm of nature is very real, but when you have been brought up without any real connection to it, you must learn to trust your perceptions of what is occurring. Once you open the door to this realm and begin to trust your senses, it becomes a magical experience. You step across a threshold and your view of the world changes forever. Every aspect of the nature realm takes on its own personality and relates to you with its own energy. You learn to recognize which devas or nature spirits are engaging you in communication by the very nature of the energy that you are perceiving.

By observation and direct experience, we have developed our ritual of preparation of the falling leaf essences. It is with the nature spirits' permission and expressed wish that I convey this information.

The devic and nature realm's desire is that we in the human realm get to know and understand that which we once knew but has been lost to today's world. It is of the utmost importance that this connection be restored to our civilization, for this is our only way of bringing back balance to not just this earth but also the entire cosmos.

We, as humans, do not have any idea of the ramifications that our actions on the earth have in relation to the rest of the cosmos. We think that we are only a small speck in the system, but consider the realm of the human body: If a small but vital part, such as the heart, becomes out of balance with the rest of the body, then does not the entire body have a big problem? The same holds true for the cosmos; when a small part becomes imbalanced, the vibration is felt on all different levels throughout the entire system.

Now is the time to start our learning and rebuild the bridge to the nature realms. I can convey this to you by relating my direct experience.

Each making of an essence carries with it a unique experience. On the day that we have chosen to collect leaves, we generally attune to the deva of the area that we intend to collect from. Through silent communication and ritual that over time we have developed, we seek permission from this deva to collect the appropriate leaves that present themselves. There has to be a trust and a relationship in existence between ourselves and the nature realm for the making of the essences to be successful. Having communicated our intentions for the day, we set out to the place we have chosen. Upon arrival, we attune ourselves to the deva of each individual tree and seek its permission and cooperation in the collection and making of the falling leaf essences. The deva in turn communicates this to the other nature spirits and elementals connected to each tree, and from this an understanding and a harmony come into being. If at any time permission is not given, it is because the deva of the tree considers that it is not the right time for collection and the making of this tree's essence, and we honor the deva's wishes. If the nature spirits and elementals feel threatened or misunderstood, we may communicate with them ourselves.

Once clear communication is established and permission is received, we collect the autumn leaves while they are actually in free fall, place them in a paper bag, and clearly label the bag.

When we have collected what we set out for, we return to the area outside the essence room where we are going to make the actual essences. We pour pure springwater into a clean glass dish and drop in the autumn leaves of a particular tree. The dish is then placed in the shade, covered, labeled, and gently rocked a number of times to emulate the motion of free fall. The essence is left for a time, rocked once more, then left to rest again. Then the leaves are removed, allowed to dry, pressed, labeled, and placed into a book for our records.

On an energetic level, the devas, nature spirits, and elementals connected to each tree cooperate in the making of the essence. This work can be very energetically demanding. In my experience, the person making the essence actually experiences some form of the essence's effects. As the essence reaches its full vibratory resonance, I, too, experience an energetic realignment and healing that tells me that the essence I am making is now complete.

We then decant the essence water into a storage bottle, and to this we add alcohol as a preservative. This solution then becomes our stock, and from it we dispense smaller bottles of essences. Once the essence is made, we store it in a place that has been created in cooperation with the nature realms. We keep an ongoing relationship with the different devas, nature spirits, and elementals to maintain a harmonious environment among the essences.

8 Using Falling Leaf Essences in Practice

THERE IS NO DOUBT THAT FALLING LEAF ESSENCES can be powerful in their action and outcome. Repeatedly, clients who have previously experienced herbs, vitamins, flower essences, and homeopathy respond to falling leaf essences in the vein of "What was *that?*" It is not that these other therapeutic substances lack power, but rather that the kind of power inherent in falling leaf essences is clearly different. But with unique power come responsibility and the need for corresponding levels of understanding. It cannot be overstated that indiscriminate or improper use of almost any kind of essence is capable of generating profound psychological and physical disturbance in susceptible people.

Generally speaking, essence therapy has eluded creeping government regulation of health care modalities in most Western countries to date. In some countries it is recognized that a person needs several years of training to practice homoeopathy to a professional standard, and thus many or even most homeopathics are available only on a practitioner basis. This appears to be a reasonable restriction, both because of the complexity of homeopathy and because these essences are capable of provoking the so-called homeopathic aggravation. In contrast, Bach flower remedies (and other flower essences) have the reputation of being fairly docile and well behaved in nature, such that in most countries they are widely available not just to practitioners but to the general public as well. There are thousands of laypeople who have Bach or other flower essence kits that they use for themselves, their families, their friends, and even their pets. These essences in lay hands certainly do a great deal of good and probably relatively little harm.

Falling leaf essences lie somewhere between flower essences and homeopathics in terms of safety and suitability for use by laypeople. I have no hesitation in recommending them to a wide range of health care professionals, including naturopaths, homeopaths, medical doctors, psychologists, kinesiologists, and massage therapists. Laypeople who have had considerable experience in using Bach or other flower essences or Schuessler cell salts may also do well with falling leaf essences. However, for novices, flower essences are a better starting point than falling leaf essences. Representing as they do the summer season of abundance and creativity, flower essences are usually gentler in their action. Also, flower essences affect the spirit and emotions more so than the physical body. Therefore, there is much less chance of provoking a physical problem through inappropriate prescribing of flower essences than there is with falling leaf essences.

Storing Your Falling Leaf Stocks

Falling leaf essence stocks are best stored away from direct sunlight and away from strong aromatic substances. Generally speaking, essences can be expected to last longer in good condition if they are stored in a wooden box that offers some ventilation. Such a box protects the essences both against the environment and against subtle energies.

Dispensing Essences

Dispensing essences is not difficult and can be presented in several steps:

1. Dispense drops from the stock bottle into a prescription bottle.

The number of drops depends on the size of the prescription bottle.

15 ml dispensing bottle: Use 2 drops of stock.

25 ml dispensing bottle: Use 3 drops of stock.

50 ml dispensing bottle: Use 5 drops of stock.

100 ml dispensing bottle: Use 7 drops of stock.

2. As few as one or as many as four falling leaf essences can be put in the one prescription bottle. Add them sequentially using the recommended number of drops for each as noted in step 1. That is, the numbers given in step 1 are for each essence (up to four essences) and not for the total number of drops of essence.

   With the exception of experienced practitioners, one should not put other essences such as tissue salts, homeopathics, and flower essences in the same bottle as falling leaf essences.

3. Add a diluting agent if you need to the essence to be preserved against microorganisms. We often use water/brandy or water/ethanol. For example, 30 percent ethanol or 30 percent brandy by volume is adequate for most prescriptive purposes. Stock should not be used at full strength, as it is 70 percent ethanol and can be uncomfortable to ingest.

4. Gently invert the prescription bottle several times to mix. Do *not* shake vigorously or bang on a surface.

5. The dosage for adults is generally in the range of 7 drops under the tongue one to four times daily. The dosage for children is less, generally proportional to body weight. A typical dose for a five-year-old would be 3 drops under the tongue once daily; for a ten-year-old, 3 drops under the tongue twice daily. Prescription of falling leaf essences for children under two years of age is best left to an experienced practitioner. Personally, I do not use them or recommend them for babies less than six months in age.

Principles for Prescription

The following principles are partly intuitive, partly the outcome of several years' experience, and partly common sense.

✿ Avoid Overuse

Do not overuse falling leaf essences. When the primary need is RELEASE AND LET GO, falling leaf essences are appropriate and excellent. However, there are other situations in which flower essences, homeopathics, herbs, vitamins, pharmaceutical's, or bodywork will outperform falling leaf essences.

In my own practice, falling leaf essences constitute no more than 15 to 20 percent of the essences I use. Why am I so sparing? It's certainly not because I am not keen or enthusiastic about them. I have an enduring respect and passion for these essences. Rather, my role as a therapist is to select that which is most appropriate to the issue or illness the client presents. Falling leaf essences, while very powerful in the areas in which they have strength, are not always the appropriate essences for a particular problem.

✿ Give It Time

A person must be given adequate time to integrate the changes that a falling leaf essence brings. Change indeed occurs in life with or without essences. An appropriate falling leaf essence brings with it an acceleration of change, allowing a person to release or let go of fear of change. Deep inner processes of release often are accompanied by a variety of feelings. There can be a sense of relief and even excitement that some old thing is passing. There can be grief and sadness. There is commonly a disorientation, a feeling of "Where am I?" and an uncertainty about what changes are needed.

If falling leaf essences are prescribed in a clinical setting with follow-up appointments, the therapist must judge whether the client has fully integrated the last falling leaf prescription before prescribing, if necessary, another. To superimpose a new falling leaf essence on an unsettled intensity resulting from the previous essence can sometimes produce an unnecessary overwhelming of the person's ability to detoxify mentally, emotionally, and physically. The general principle is not to prescribe another falling leaf essence if there is uncertainty as to whether the previous essence is still affecting a person. Instead, the therapist might consider a gently supportive flower essence or gem elixir.

In my own experience with falling leaf essences, I most commonly prescribe only once. On occasion I prescribe twice in succession within several weeks. Very rarely have I made three successive prescriptions, and only then with clients who clearly were integrating the changes easily and well.

✿ Prescribe for the Issues That Present

Falling leaf essences should be prescribed on the basis of the issues that are currently presenting in a person's life. If we were to look through the list of 160 falling leaf essences described in chapter 5, we might all decide that we need 120+ of them! For example, each of us would benefit from releasing anger, hatred, or our feelings about past relationships. In theory, we could all benefit from those falling leaf essences that pertain to the liver, kidneys, and lymphatics for detoxification of the physical body.

However, the need for releasing and letting go is ongoing in life and may be represented like the layers of an onion. With an onion, one begins by peeling off the outermost layer, that which is currently visible. So it is with people; their current awareness is the outer onion skin layer that needs to be peeled off first. It would indeed be extraordinarily difficult to peel an onion beginning with the tenth innermost layer! A falling leaf prescription aimed at an inner layer is quite inappropriate and can cause needless difficulty and stress. People are ready and usually able to deal with issues that are already beginning to present in their awareness. They are usually not ready and sometimes unable to deal with submerged issues that haven't surfaced yet.

✿ Begin with Single Essences

Experienced falling leaf practitioners sometimes prescribe two, three, or even four falling leaf essences simultaneously, combining them in one bottle. However, one builds confidence initially by using single essences.

✿ Keep Records

Keep an organized, written record that includes the person's name, the date of prescription, the essence(s) used, and any feedback subsequently given. Such an organized record of prescriptions and results is invaluable in building one's confidence. One is also able to look back over this record at any time, which can enable one to ascertain the effectiveness of one's prescriptions and make any needed changes to one's prescribing habits.

⚘ Don't Force a Prescription

Prescribe an essence only if the person really wants it. A falling leaf essence can be offered but not inflicted. A reluctant client may subconsciously block or resist the essence from the outset. In my experience, falling leaf essences are much more difficult to obstruct than flower essences. They have a tenacity and physicality about their action that makes them almost irresistible. Nevertheless, introducing a falling leaf essence into a resistant and skeptical environment is not always the path of wisdom.

⚘ Be Cautious

Use caution when prescribing for the very young, the very elderly, and the physically or psychologically impaired. These categories of people all have limited or impaired abilities to detoxify, to let go, or to release. I do not used falling leaf essences at all with infants of less than six months of age. With children over the age of six months, a dosage much lower than that prescribed for adults is appropriate. Sometimes that dosage can be just 1 or 2 drops daily.

Falling leaf essences have a stronger action when given orally than when the drops are placed on the wrist and allowed to absorb through the skin. A valid option for those who may be hypersensitive to a falling leaf essence is to place 1 drop on the wrist daily, allowing to dry. I recall one or two cases where a single drop administered in this way every second or third day proved sufficient for an action of the remedy.

An alternative approach for infants is to administer the falling leaf essence to the mother. Because of the very strong energetic and physical bond of mother and child, an essence administered to the mother will also act on the child, but in a buffered or attenuated way. Bear in mind that if the mother is still breastfeeding the baby, the essence will come across more directly to the baby via the breast milk.

Elderly people and those with serious debilitating disease usually have less ability to change and more difficulty on a bodily level in achieving the desired detoxification. It is generally helpful to examine elderly people on a case-by-case basis. Some elderly people are quite robust and might do well with falling leaf essences. Others are frail and delicate in appearance, and they should not use falling leaf essences.

If one is concerned as to whether an individual is too weak or hypersensitive for falling leaf essences, a valid approach is to begin with a low dosage. Give just 1 drop daily, increasing gradually only if all proceeds well.

ᚙ Interact with the Intended Recipient

Falling leaf essences generally work best if their prescription arises out of interaction with a person. The act of verbalization brings an issue to a point of greater accessibility within a person's being. Indeed, counselors and psychologists are well aware that the simple act of expressing an issue before an empathetic practitioner can itself trigger significant catharsis or release. An essence will work to its best potential when the person is working with it—that is, when the person is aware of the issues or emotions that the essence is intended to address. The person's conscious involvement complements the essence's transformative abilities.

ᚙ Develop a Personal Philosophy

Practitioners must each develop their own way of using the essence that is consistent with their own philosophy of healing. It is a very useful exercise for healers to write down what they seek to accomplish in their healing work. The more specific they can be, the better. For example, the goal to "heal people on all levels" is too general and vague to be of much use. By contrast, the goal to help people release issues, memories, and emotions from the past that hold them back or inhibit their potential in the present is clear and good. Working from this foundational statement, one can then select appropriate groups of essences to work with and also appropriate ways of using the essences.

Supplements to Falling Leaf Essences

There are a number of natural substances that appear to increase the strength of action of falling leaf essences. Mineral supplements, ginseng, noni juice, certain B-complex vitamins, and the algae chlorella and spirulina are among them. In my own experience, these supplements are of limited value, because the action of falling leaf essences in standard dosage is already strong enough. More often I need to reduce the dosage than to think of ways of increasing the action. However, other practitioners find these supplements helpful.

The Practitioner-Client Relationship

When falling leaf essences exist in the context of the practitioner-client relationship, the nature of that relationship becomes important. Diagram 8.1 illustrates the triangle of energy that exists in prescriptive essence therapy. In order for the remedy to have good action, energy must be able to flow unimpeded around the triangle. Clearly, blockages in energy flow can occur at several points in the triangle. Practitioners are generally aware of the capability of their clients to potentially obstruct the action of essences. Such obstruction can occur at a subconscious level for a variety of reasons. However, as diagram 8.1 illustrates, blockage in energy flow can also occur at the level of the practitioner. That is, if practitioners are themselves obstructed in the action area of the essence they are prescribing, they can become an obstacle.

When an essence prescription proves ineffective, practitioners often seek assistance and understanding as to why. In such situations, practitioners are usually aware of the possibility of the client blocking the essence. Rarely have they considered the possibility that their own life experience might be sufficiently obstructed in the area of prescription to effectively block the action of the essence.

Another possibility is blockage at the level of the essence. As a conscious, intelligent, noncellular being, an essence is capable of contributing energy into a situation or of withdrawing its energy. The essence is like a worker assigned a task. The worker might decide to go

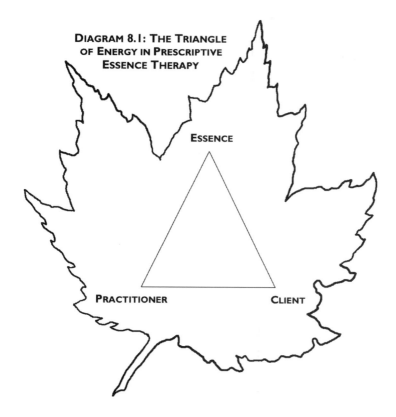

DIAGRAM 8.1: THE TRIANGLE
OF ENERGY IN PRESCRIPTIVE
ESSENCE THERAPY

ESSENCE

PRACTITIONER   CLIENT

ahead with the task wholeheartedly or with partial commitment or to leave the task completely. This is perhaps the most mysterious and least understood aspect of the situation. Who can understand or plumb the depths of the psyche of an immaterial essence? Perhaps an essence becomes unwilling to contribute its energy when the person taking it is insincere about seeking change or is seeking to use the essence to support rather than change dysfunctional patterns.

An important aspect of diagram 8.1 is the energetic connection between the practitioner and the client. There is nothing more undermining to the action of an essence than the intrusion of games into the practitioner-client relationship. *Games* may be defined as any aspects of the interaction, conscious or unconscious, which are not both honest and direct. Thus, by definition, games are either not honest or truthful, or they are indirect, or both. Games represent a subconscious collusion between practitioner and client to block or attenuate the action of an essence and as such represent the most potent means of sabotage of an essence's action. Eric Berne has described in detail and with humor the common kinds of games that people play in the context of life in general.[1] Practitioner-client games could be identified and named in a similar vein. These might include, from the practitioner's viewpoint, "I'm good enough to fix you," "Just take my advice and you'll be okay," and "You've come to the right place." Common client games include "I just need sympathy and support," "Please be my hero," and "I need both my illness and therapy." Games may be initiated by practitioner or client, but it always takes two to sustain a game. Such games inevitably result in a reduced action of the essence. A straightjacket from the outset.

The Therapist's Qualifications

It is obvious from the considerations discussed above that the primary qualification for being a falling leaf essence therapist is to have a good movement or flow in one's own life experience. If one has major obstructions in one's own life, these obstructions will severely restrict the flow of energy in diagram 8.1. That is, one must have a deep, ongoing commitment to one's own personal growth process to be suitable as a falling leaf essence therapist. Note that this primary qualification is experiential, not academic. One could in principle pass with high honors written examinations about falling leaf essences but be quite unsuitable and unsatisfactory as a practitioner. As the adage goes, "Walk the talk." A practitioner needs to be in an appropriate state not just mentally but also spiritually, emotionally, and physically.

Practitioner Testimonials

Several practitioners have joined me in using falling leaf essences over the past several years. They each have their own approach to healing and have developed their own perspective on falling leaf essences. Their testimonials follow.

Please note that no claims can be made concerning the ability of falling leaf essences to cure any medical conditions. Practitioners may report that in a particular instance, a client with condition X improved while taking falling leaf essence Y. The improvement may be the result of the falling leaf essence, it may be a fluctuation in the condition that would have occurred without the essence, or it may even be the result of some other therapy that the person was undergoing without the therapist's knowledge. Even if the improvement can be attributed to the action of a falling leaf essence, there is no justification in extrapolating from one case of condition X to condition X in general. It is such generalization and unjustified claims of effectiveness for natural remedies that have long exposed such remedies to well-justified criticism.

⚘ Libby Gordon

Libby Gordon is a busy therapist who works with both bodywork and essences.

I have a therapy practice in a little suburb called Hartwell, Victoria. I share this clinic with my sister and a medical practitioner, and we call it Heartwell Healing Centre. The name signifies our focus; it is through the "heart" element of healing that we endeavor to reach and help the clients who come through our door.

Our journey into healing began over twenty years ago when I dared to ask the inner question "Is this all there is?" I began working with Reiki and progressed from this point. Interestingly, I had always been drawn to the use of flower essences, in particular the wonderful elixir Rescue Remedy. I was a strong believer in this magnificent essence, and throughout my early years of parenting it was never out of reach. Many, many times this essence came to my "rescue," both for my children and for myself.

When two of my children were still very young, I happened to wander with them into the office of a flower essence practitioner in my area. She was also an illustrator of children's books, and I was fascinated with the life-sized murals of fairies, elves, and nature spirits that were spread all over her walls. As we roamed her studio, she offered to do an essence "reading" for me and my children. I agreed. The results of the reading of my three-year-old daughter were startling. The practitioner told me that she needed the flower essence Zinnia, which is recommended for helping people remember the child in themselves. It is usually given to adults—certainly not to a three-year-old. When the practitioner brought this to my attention, she asked if my daughter was serious and whether she rarely laughed. I told her that yes, my daughter was indeed very serious.

I agreed to allow my daughter to take Zinnia, and the practitioner warned me this could have some repercussions. It did not take long for the warning to come true. That night my daughter experienced a major healing crisis. It was a very long night for me as I lay in her bed and cuddled her. But to my joy, I heard her laughing within forty-eight hours, and thereafter her personality lightened up considerably.

Flower essences then proceeded to become an even more important part of my life. I traveled eventually through the world of aromatherapy, other bodywork modalities, and numerous counseling techniques. And my essence work grew and grew.

For many years I enjoyed using the Australian Bush flower essences. I felt particularly attached to these lovely and highly beneficial healing essences. However, there is an old saying that holds a lot of power: "When the student is ready, the teacher appears." For me, that teacher was Grant Lambert.

When Grant and I met, we realized we had something to offer each other and proceeded to work together. I explored his essences and gradually expanded my repertoire. I am fortunate enough to have a very busy clinical practice that offers remedial bodywork, counseling, self-help techniques, and, of course, essences. With this busy clientele, I had a ready-made market with which to research these unknown essences.

I may work differently from other practitioners in this field, because I use Grant's essences as a "guidebook." I first ask silent permission to be in touch with the client's highest self. After making sure I am centered and as clear as possible, with the aid of my intuition, I ask to be shown what the client needs. Generally, two or three essences will be chosen intuitively that then open doorways to an understanding of the client's presenting challenge. With this information and the aid of a few minutes of questioning, an in-depth picture of the client's core issues will present themselves.

For example, a client may present with endometriosis, which is a challenging pathology to work with. After having checked her medical history, drug usage, and treatments to date, it is important to ascertain which is the "body"—spiritual, mental, emotional, or physical—that is predominantly holding the challenge of this condition. I would also ascertain whether supporting modalities such as naturopathy, herbal medicine, homeopathy, and bodywork need to be combined with the essence therapy. I then ask to be given the conscious or unconscious fears associated with the condition. In many instances, this condition is attached to lack of feminine nurturing or fear of intimacy. The falling leaf essences very often form the core of the therapeutic picture which emerges.

If her presenting condition is affected predominantly (say 60 percent) by her emotional body, the essences Weeping Katsura Tree (FLE 17; release fear of love) or Burr Oak (FLE 111; release fear of inadequacy) along with Weeping Elm (FLE 44; release emotional turmoil) may be selected. After sharing with the client what I am learning, I question her as to whether the information resonates with her. If more accurate descriptions are needed, we then proceed to "peel away the onion layers" as they present. At all times the client is in charge. I see my role as gently opening doorways of possibilities so that the client can "heal herself" to the best of her ability.

I find that essences, in conjunction with bodywork when appropriate, gently open the client to healing unconscious wounds. Obviously no two clients are the same. Some may require a good deal of assistance, while others have a very clear understanding of their journey and through their dreams or writing or inner work come to a healing conclusion through their own resources.

Without a doubt, the practice of using essences skillfully is in asking the "right" questions and in having *no attachment* to the outcome of the answers given.

Over the past year, I have found that Oriental Plane (FLE 16; release fear of change) has been of great use in my practice. Our reality on this vast planet is ever changing at a rapid pace, and there appears to be more and more chaos on both a macrocosmic and a microcosmic level. As human beings, one of the realities we fear most is "change," as it evades our control while having such great impact on our lives. The reality is, too, that most of us can cope with change only in small doses. I have used Oriental Plane extensively in my practice, with wonderful results. It enables people to remove the fear of the "what ifs," helping them focus their energy on coping with daily living and not dwell so much in the future of the "what ifs." Of course, fear of change can mean many things to many people, and what is frightening for one client may be inconsequential to another. It is important to remember the client's perspective and to honor each reality.

The falling leaf family of essences ranges far and wide in its power to cope with a huge variety of presenting conditions. My case histories are in their hundreds and very varied, and it feels almost like cheating to isolate one or two as an example. Instead, I'd like to note some of the essences that seem to arise most frequently for my clients. They include African Laburnum (FLE 138; skin problems), Apricot (FLE 14; release anger), Japanese Maple (FLE 87; irritable bowel), Oriental Plane (FLE 16; release fear of change), Silver Birch (FLE 31; release struggle), Trident Maple (FLE 77; anxiety), and Turkistan Birch (FLE 130; release persistent anxiety).

The combination and complex essences are a wonderful tool for anyone in clinical practice, no matter what the modality. They are easy to use and usually self-explanatory. I have a large freestanding glass cabinet in my reception area and while the clients are waiting for their appointment, it is easy for them to peruse the combination and complex essences. As the explanation cards are written clearly, choices are either very easy or difficult—difficult because the common response is: "I feel I need nearly half these essences; how many am I allowed to have?"

The results are fast, powerful, and most effective. What appeals to me most is the self-empowerment clients can feel as they take responsibility for choosing a healing remedy for themselves instead of the practitioner presenting choices to them.

The most common combination essences that are selected are: Shock and Trauma Remedy, Fear of the Unknown, Emotional Wellbeing, Anti-*Candida*, Becoming Your Own Person, and Release Control.

These essences do not have a "sledgehammer" effect but, rather, inspire the gradual awakening of realization to the conscious or unconscious challenge being presented. I feel most privileged to have such a wonderful repertoire of healing essences in my practice.

✿ Lee Jackson

Lee Jackson is an enthusiastic therapist, whose interests range from bodywork and essences to working with earth energies.

I have been working with falling leaf essences for three years now, and in that time I have experienced an enormous amount of growth in myself. When I first began using these essences, it felt as though people were not quite ready for them, and distrust was commonplace. But as the earth's energy systems change and new challenges occur in families, the workplace, and individuals, people's acceptance level has, I have found, slowly increased.

My practice also includes Reiki/Sechiem, earth acupuncture, and dowsing. These modalities complement one another as an energetic release system. They begin in the home or working environment, clearing negative energies, and follow through to personal emotional and mental problems, releasing them with the use of falling leaf essences, counseling, or Reiki as needed.

The dispensing of falling leaf essences is not just mixing the essence and handing over the bottle. For me it is a spiritual acknowledgment. Holding the client's problem in my mind, I gently invert the bottle (usually five times), forming a connection triangle between God, the essence, and myself. This inversion is what makes the essence unique for me; it is an honoring of the tree, the leaf, and the release it gives. It is also a parting of the way; the essence is released with love, knowing it is fulfilling its life's purpose as a healing modality. This process occurs naturally in me, as I connect at a heart level with the essences. I don't believe it changes the vibration of the essence, but it enhances the essence with my own vibration. I believe that each practitioner, when dispensing the essence, will bring to it his or her own personal essence of self.

A simple case was when I recommended to an elderly gentleman the essence Trident Maple (FLE 77; anxiety). He was leaving his home of forty years to retire to a small apartment, and he was feeling anxious. About four weeks later he rang back to get another bottle of the essence. He said that he had never slept so well. It was wonderful to hear he was sleeping so soundly, but I inquired as to why he still needed the essence. Apparently he had been a milkman all his adult life and had only ever had four hours' sleep a night. I concluded that his body clock was ready to retire, but his conditional patterning was causing the anxiety. I recommended the falling leaf essence Silver Birch (FLE 31; release struggle) with a dosage of 4 drops twice daily. He rang back a couple of days later to say that it was making him more anxious. This was the release coming through; the nature of the essence can cause discomfort. I dropped the dosage down to 2 drops twice daily and gave him another bottle of Trident Maple; he took both and is now settling into retirement.

In another case, I was dowsing a client's home for negative buildup of energies in the lounge room. The house had been built in the late 1800s, and the natural flow of energy under the house had blocked up, allowing negative energies to collect and causing disturbing emotional behaviors in the house. The last two owners of the house had sold it due to marriage breakups, and my client's previous relationship had ended in the lounge room. I cleared unfavorable earth energies under his house using earth acupuncture and treated the client with Red Crepe Myrtle (FLE 38; release possessiveness). The essence helped him release his own negative energies.

Another case I would like to share is that of a lady who came to me with stress-related work problems. She had not been able to take any time for herself and had been working late shifts to earn enough money to pay off a large debt. This woman had been on a spiritual path for some time but had lost sight of those connections. Because she expended so much energy worrying about the payments, her creative drive had dried up, and she felt stressed and overworked. I recommended Glory Vine (FLE 22; release mental control) to help her remove the boundaries created by the mind. This essence helped her perceive her life from the realm of spiritual feeling rather than physical thought, allowing her more energy for her spiritual journey. She was still able to work toward paying off the debt, but she now also felt the desire to regain her spiritual teaching skills. Her creative flow is now enhancing her life.

There are certain essences I use with people to give an initial sense of trust in life and in the processes of the free-fall change that it takes us through, an ability that is unique to the falling leaf essences. Cherry Plum (FLE 7; emotional well-being), Linden (FLE 2; tonic), and Trident Maple (FLE 77; anxiety) are the three main essences I use for this purpose. These three essences are also useful for calming nervous tension, promoting general well-being, and giving that extra boost when needed.

I find that I have integrated the overall essence of falling leaf essences through my work with them as a practitioner. I have not only helped clients but also worked through and released an enormous amount of my own blocks and control patterns. These essences have brought about a balance in me and continue to do so, and they have instilled in me an incredible trust in the flow of life. People and experiences are presented to me at just the right moment to bring in the change; the essence helps in the release, bringing about a calmness and strength in me as I live life to my fullest potential.

✍ *Robyn Wood*

Robyn Wood is a practitioner who uses a variety of healing modalities. Robyn lives and works in idyllic surroundings near Olinda in the Dandenongs near Melbourne.

Over the years in my work as a natural therapist, it has become increasingly clear to me that working with just one modality is very limiting and certainly does not accommodate the needs of all people. To provide the optimum treatment, I have found it important to have several tools in the practitioner tool kit that can be drawn upon to suit a particular client's need. It is common practice for me to offer essences as an adjunct to whatever other treatment may be administered on the day. I find these wonderfully complementary and was delighted to be one of the practitioners to trial the falling leaf essences before their release to the public.

An illustration of how I work with the essences in consultation with clients follows.

Clients are usually able to express why they have come. If this is not the case, it soon becomes clear as the interaction continues. Most commonly, clients present with physical pain in some part of the body, with some kind of organic imbalance, or with emotional distress about a particular issue. Within the first minutes, I silently make an invocation to the divine healing energies, surrendering to their guidance and asking what would be the most appropriate treatment for the highest good of the client at this time. A clear response is typically quite immediate. The direction may be Bowen therapy (type of bodywork developed by Australian Tom Bowen), pranic healing, cutting the ties that bind, or counseling. If at all in doubt, I will then dowse to clarify my perception.

Regardless of which modality is chosen for the client, at some stage in the consultation or toward the end, I quietly ask the divine healing energies, "Is it wisdom for this person to have essences at this time?" My experience has been that only a rare few clients do not require essences with either the first or the second visit. There are also the occasions when I feel no treatment is needed except for essences. This is typical for clients who need some support for the physical body or assistance in dealing with a specific issue they are working through. An example would be someone who is processing a relationship breakdown. A possible essence for this situation might be European Pussy Willow (FLE 80; depression), Peach (FLE 71; personal growth), Trident Maple (FLE 77; anxiety), or White Flowering Plum (FLE 72; let go of a relationship).

Very early in my practice as a natural therapist I was drawn to the Bush flower essences and those of ancient civilizations. Now I use these essences only in a limited manner. I find it intriguing that falling leaf essences seem to have supplanted these other essences. There so often seems to be one or more falling leaf essences that is most appropriate for my own personal use as well as for friends, family, and clients. "What about my investment in all the other essences?" I pondered.

Over time I have reflected about the possible factors influencing this situation. I have realized that my energy resonates very well with tree energy, which is likely enhanced by the fact that both my home and my practice are in the Dandenongs, a very beautiful and heavily treed area in the outer suburbs of Melbourne. Another realization is that I myself have had the need to let go of a lot of issues; hence I seem to have attracted people who have needed to do the same. These are often the same people who attend personal growth classes I conduct, the core content of which is about letting go and moving on.

While the universe will no doubt continue to provide others and myself the opportunities for further spiritual growth, I'm aware of a deepening sense of surrender, calm, and connection to all that is. There is no doubt in my mind that the falling leaf essences have been a major contributor to this state.

In the following case histories, for reasons of confidentiality I have changed the names of my clients.

Owen had a fall from his motorcycle three weeks prior to seeing me. He presented with left hip pain, and the left thigh was very swollen. Back and shoulder pain was less by comparison. He had been seeing his local doctor two or three times a week since the accident to drain the fluid from his thigh, and he was taking anti-inflammatories orally. There was little to no improvement of his overall condition throughout this treatment.

My first consultation with Owen consisted of Neuro-Structural Integration Technique (NST; a form of Bowen therapy) to rebalance the body and address the specific areas of pain. Preceding that was a few minutes of pranic healing to give a quick clean to the human energy field. I also recommended that Owen apply a compress of washing soda below the thigh overnight to assist the drainage. A few days later Owen reported less hip pain, but his leg was still very swollen.

A week later the second treatment was a repeat of the pranic healing and NST treatment. I gave Owen some falling leaf essences to take orally: Pink Horse Chestnut (FLE 13; fluid retention), Liquidamber (FLE 10; inflammation), and Judas Tree (FLE 148; lymphatic cleansing). I told him to take 7 drops of the essences given together in one bottle every hour for 24 hours, and thereafter three times a day. Three days later Owen claimed a dramatic improvement. The swelling had reduced and the hip pain was only moderate. Following the third and final treatment, Owen reported that he "felt great," and the presenting problem was totally resolved.

Jane's twenty-eight-year-old daughter had died from a drug overdose six months prior to our initial consultation. At first Jane had coped reasonably well, but recently she had become very depressed and unable to talk about her grief. Although her doctor recommended counseling, that didn't feel right for Jane. During our initial consultation,

I suggested the process of cutting the ties that bind, a method that taps into the subconscious through the use of symbology. Jane responded favorably, and we set up a process by means of which she would energetically disconnect from dysfunctional ties with her deceased daughter. Her homework was to work with a figure-eight symbol each day for two weeks. In addition I gave Jane Dove Tree (FLE 3; bereavement) to be taken three times daily. Within three or four days, Jane reported that she felt the essence working, and then she came down with flulike symptoms. Upon her return consultation two weeks later to complete the cut, Jane shared that once she had recovered from the illness, she felt very peaceful, knowing that something had shifted significantly. To further support her transition, I gave her Persian Witch Hazel (FLE 27; release children).

Mary called me from a psychiatric hospital where she had been placed with severe postnatal depression after the difficult birth of her firstborn child, a son who was then six weeks old. There were no apparent physical dysfunctions for either Mary or her baby. Mary's husband and mother were very supportive, but nevertheless she felt unable to cope and was fearful of being alone with her son. Confusion also prevailed because she didn't want to stay in the hospital but was deeply concerned about returning home and taking on the responsibilities of motherhood.

The new father delivered his wife and son to my door for their first consultation. Pranic healing was the treatment for both, in addition to just a few moves of Bowen therapy for the baby, I gave Mary a combination of Oriental Plane (FLE 16; release fear of change), European Pussy Willow (FLE 80; depression), and Turkistan Birch (FLE 130; release persistent anxiety). The dosage was 7 drops every hour for 24 hours and thereafter three times a day. For the baby, I gave Mary Bush flower essences to be added to his daily bath and applied topically to the forehead twice a day. Mother and baby returned for a second treatment of pranic healing a few days later, and Mary returned on her own for two subsequent treatments in the following week. She then felt confident to return home and care for her son with the loving support of her mother and her husband.

My experience with falling leaf essences has been an incredible journey. The essences I most commonly administer are Cherry Plum (FLE 7; emotional well-being), European Pussy Willow (FLE 80; depression), Pin Oak (FLE 8; fatigue), Silver Birch (FLE 31; release struggle), Trident Maple (FLE 77; anxiety), and White Flowering Plum (FLE 72; let go of a relationship). During the last six months, I have found the essence Oriental Plane (FLE 16; release fear of change) also to be in great demand.

Even my dear canine friends and companions Harley and Rose, who were both born with heart conditions, have benefited greatly from falling leaf essences, particularly Tulip Tree (FLE 26; heart). Regular consultations for my pets with a veterinarian who prefers to work with natural therapies show no apparent signs of heart deterioration; the veterinarian has commented on the dogs' vitality, particularly as they are now approaching the end of their expected life span. I confided with her that I had been giving them Crab Apple (FLE 53; elixir of youth) in recent months and had noticed an increase in playfulness. Harley and Rose have been willing recipients of several other falling leaf essences. I have given them Eastern Red Bud (FLE 95; release fear of abandonment) when they board with friends and have given Spice Bush (FLE 124; obsessive behaviors) to Harley to reduce continual licking.

Though I use falling leaf essences primarily to enhance whatever other treatment I may provide, it would be presumptuous to suggest that they have a subordinate role. I have come to view these essences as vibrational energies that afford great respect. They may take only a few minutes to prepare, but they are the most important aspect of the treatment and sometimes are the stimulus for the greatest transformation in the well-being of the recipient. My experience has been that they are incredibly powerful and an amazing healing tool.

Author's Note: In recent times, Robyn Wood has been exploring the potential of essences described in this book, particularly falling leaf essences, snow-modified Australian flower essences, and bark essences, in feng shui. The idea here is that an essence bottle placed appropriately within a room or dwelling, is capable of favorably altering the flow of energy. Since an essence has a subtle energetic field that extends far beyond the containing bottle, it is able to alter the surrounding energy. This can be used in addition to, or instead of, traditional feng shui solutions. Robyn has had considerable success with the essence approach to feng shui.

❧ Randolph Toombs

Randolph was born in Philadelphia. His area of particular interest lies in alternative and vibrational medicine. In 1993 he established the Healing Hands Massage Clinic on the island of Tasmania, off the southern coast of Australia.

On the healing island of Tasmania, Australia, which straddles the Pacific and Indian Oceans, sits the North Hobart site of the Healing Hands Massage Clinic. Here we're aware of the interdependence of all the human faculties; we understand that gentle touch and deep tissue massage are only Band-Aid treatments for life's stresses.

Bodywork practitioners know well the presenting symptoms appearing in stress, insomnia, headaches and migraines, strains and sprains, torticollis (stiff, sore, "noisy" neck), sinusitis, lymphatic congestion, sore ankles, inflexible knees and hips, tennis elbow, foot disorders, shinsplints, "frozen shoulder," sciatica, dowager's hump, scarring from lumbar and cervical spinal fusion operations, postoperative adhesions, *Polymyalgia rheumatica,* arthritis, and paralysis. All too often the assumption is that bodywork is all that's needed; never mind the causal factors to be found in the four human faculties.

Human faculties are interlinked in a pyramid. At the top of the pyramid sits our spirit, which is linked to a higher consciousness ("God"). Through this spiritual connection, many as children obtain spiritual light, love, truth, justice, joy, peace, and harmony—hence the innocence, resilience, trust, and delightfulness of young children. However, let there be repeated pain experienced in the course of life and loss, and the developing mind, stimulated by fear, begins to interfere with spirit.

Undisturbed, our spirit would interface with parts of the human mind and develop the sixteen psychic faculties (identified by the research of Dr. J. V. Rhine of Duke University in his book *Clock Without Hands*), imbuing us with everything from telepathy to creativity. Break the link between spirit and the psychic and our awareness is trapped in three-dimensional physicality and linear time. We refer to this as "growing up" and leaving behind "the imaginary."

Now the symptoms of disconnection from our spiritual source migrate down to the emotional faculty, where, unless we have a loving home environment, we experience anxiety and adolescent depression. Our hang-ups begin.

Our presumptuous forebrain and left hemisphere begin to dominate our awareness.

Finally our body manifests the imbalance; and we recognize that "there is a problem." Now we ask the practitioner for a quick fix.

Quantum physics informs us that all the human faculties are energy at different vibrational frequencies. Thus there is the need for "vibrational medicine" such as falling leaf essences to complement conventional medicine and massage and to restore the natural balance. The natural balance of our faculties can be disturbed, leaving us with unhealthy hang-ups and habits that we later call parts of our character. These can keep us from fulfilling our life's potential. Releasing them used to be an expensive, painstaking experience. With the use of Dr. Grant Lambert's arboreal essences, vibrational blockages are released like the falling of leaves.

Below are some of the testimonies of Randolph Toombs's clients, which he has helped them express, written in the first person. Please note that "I" refers to the client.

I have smoked thirty cigarettes per day for the past twenty-seven years. Past unsuccessful attempts at quitting have included the "cold turkey" method, nicotine chewing gum, nicotine patches, and a combination of the herbs dong quai and guarana. In the throes of my last faltering attempt to give up smoking, I was trembling, irritable, and overeating.

Then I heard about the falling leaf essence Spice Bush (FLE 124; obsessive behaviors), which treats the habit at the causal level, not just the symptomatic. Within two hours of taking the essence dosage, not only did I stop trembling, but when my wife smoked in the car while I was driving, I had not the least craving for a cigarette.

I would caution those considering this successful treatment not to become overconfident and stop taking drops before the end of the recommended three-month period.

My experience of change was as a result of taking White Ash (FLE 9; osteoarthritis). As a result of adolescent kyphosis of my thoracic spine, by the age of fifty-five, I was the bane of chiropractors and masseurs alike. Upon examining my X rays, several chiropractors would note the disk degeneration, vertebral lipping, and joint immobility and predict no better treatment outcome than the prevention of further degeneration. "Definitely no movement would occur in the spinal joints as a result of chiropractic manipulation," they would advise.

At that stage I experienced almost constant back pain that was exacerbated by walking. My footfall would send shock waves up the skeleton to the spine, pinching my nerves and further tightening my muscles. After I'd been taking White Ash for a month and wished to test for results, I asked a chiropractor to proceed with the manipulation. To our surprise, each manipulation resulted in my spinal joints freely moving, and I now can walk three hours and do one hundred situps nonstop without pain.

When one of my clients heard of such impressive results, she began taking Trident Maple (FLE 77; anxiety) to help ease her chronic anxiety. Two days after she'd begun to take the remedy, she rang me to say that on the previous night she'd noticed that the next-door neighbor's house had been burgled and vandalized and was now cordoned off by police, some of whom were searching the neighborhood for the offender. She told me that her normal reaction to such an event would have been to dash out to her car and make a getaway herself, not soon to return. Instead, she cooked herself a meal, ate it, and retired to bed for a sound night's sleep. This behavior was so uncharacteristic for her that she later reported it to me in a testimonial letter.

Another testimonial letter attests to the efficacy of Snake Bark (FLE 144; blood pressure). It reads, "My blood pressure has been high for the last four years. Walking up stairs left me breathless. By April 1999 my readings were considered dangerously high. My doctor prescribed the drugs Tritace, Plendil, and Naturlix. Yet my blood pressure readings came down only slightly and slowly. On April 19, 1999, I began taking the FLE 144. Two days later my readings had fallen to 185/110 mm/Hg. By April 29, my blood pressure had fallen to 145/95 mm/Hg. [Normal blood pressure is approximately 140/80 mm/Hg.]

As if to illustrate that it was the falling leaf essences that lowered my blood pressure, on the weekend that I ran out of Dr. Lambert's remedy and took only the medically prescribed drugs, my blood pressure rose to 160/95 mm/Hg.

I had a horseback-riding accident and consequently visited the massage clinic with pain in my right shoulder and upper back. Up until that time, the diagnosis resulting from X-ray testing was that my right ribs were out of alignment. Despite chiropractic treatment, I still had pain.

After three deep tissue massages, I began taking Pussy Willow (FLE 66; back). After I completed taking the remedy, I can honestly say all traces of pain were gone and have yet to return.

I have experienced sleep apnea, insomnia, and snoring for the past two and half years, ever since I began taking the medically prescribed drug Rohypnol. Within three days of taking Dr. Lambert's Cockspur Hawthorn (FLE 84; snoring), these three conditions ceased, and I can have eight hours of uninterrupted sleep in spite of the fact that I have continued with the drug and am a cigarette smoker.

Falling leaf essences are also beneficial in the emotional realm. One client states: "When my partner announced that he was engaged to marry another woman, I felt that without his love my life was not worth much and threatened and unsuccessfully attempted suicide. When professional help was sought by myself, I was not in the mood to accept wise counsel. I did, however, accept the falling leaf essence White Flowering Plum (FLE 72; let go of a relationship). Early the next morning, eight hours after my last dose of this remedy, the self-destructive feelings were overwhelming. Within twenty minutes of restarting the remedy, I was rationally in control again, making preparations to begin my life anew, partner or not. The remedy certainly got me through the crisis period without the side effects of antidepressants."

I revisit the three and half years in which I experienced unbearable neck and back pain and was on the medical round-about. My condition was given all sorts of Greek names—scoliosis, spondylitis, and kyphosis—and I was given everything from the usual painkillers and antidepressants to radiation therapy on the offending nerve that aggravated my condition.

I was constantly bedridden, could manage only four hours of interrupted sleep per week, could eat only my favorite food (peanut butter), was on numerous painkillers, and had cold hands and feet, difficulty breathing, anxiety attacks, and fainting. After three months of treatment consisting of deep tissue massage and Pussy Willow (FLE 66; back), White Ash (FLE 9; osteoarthritis), Willow Pattern Tree (FLE 12; nervous insomnia), Scarlet Oak (FLE 150; shoulder problems), Trident Maple (FLE 77; anxiety), and appropriate nutrient supplements, I have been able to drive a car for three hours, sleep for seven hours nightly, eat most foods, get off all but one analgesic, have normal temperature in my extremities, have no breathing difficulty, and have not reexperienced anxiety disorders or fainting.

᠗ Ruth Scolyer

Ruth Scolyer is a well-known naturopath who for several decades has lived and worked in northern Tasmania. Ruth comes from a family of herbalists, not necessarily with formal training but with an innate sense of nature and its benefits to human health. Ruth's father and grandfather both took an interest in herbal medicine, and Ruth herself has been a practicing naturopath for forty years. She ran a health foods store from 1958 until just recently. Her testimonial, as given here, arises from an interview given to Jennie Richardson.

Ruth met Grant Lambert through their shared interest in natural medicine, and they developed a good working relationship. When Grant created the falling leaf essences, Ruth was naturally one of the practitioners asked to research them. She has now been working with these essences for the past five years, and with her busy practice she has had a lot of valuable experience with them.

She has found over time that a handful of falling leaf essences regularly present for use, including Cherry Plum (FLE 7; emotional well-being), Manchurian Pear (FLE 92; release grief), Mexican Hawthorn (FLE 51; death), Pin Oak (FLE 8; fatigue), Star Magnolia (FLE 70; rheumatoid arthritis), and White Ash (FLE 9; osteoarthritis).

Because she is a naturopath, Ruth tends to use herbal medicine, homeopathic drops, and essences in her practice. She has many times combined all three with successful results. Her approach to healing is born out of the belief that when a client presents with a problem, the healer must treat the whole person. She finds that homeopathic drops and falling leaf essences, when combined, work like a bushfire—the homeopathic drops work from the physical body out to the emotional, and the falling leaf essences working from the energy field into the physical.

Ruth has also achieved excellent results using noni juice in conjunction with falling leaf essences.

A twenty-five-year-old woman with malignant tumors in her breast came to see Ruth, who gave her an herbal medicine, falling leaf essences, and two snow-modified Australian flower essences. The woman took these for six weeks, and when doctors then performed a biopsy, they found two empty sacs where the tumors had been.

Another young woman who had four children under five years of age came to see Ruth. She was very depressed and was threatening to commit suicide. Ruth asked her to think about her children and gave her an herbal remedy and Manchurian Pear (FLE 92; release grief) and European Pussy Willow (FLE 80; depression) to take for two weeks. She agreed to this. Within ten days the woman rang Ruth back. She was ready to get on with her life and could not believe the condition she had been in.

In another case, two young sisters whose parents had separated needed some support to get through their school exams. Ruth gave them Manchurian Pear (FLE 92; release grief) and Crepe Myrtle (FLE 41; uncertainty) with excellent results.

In conclusion, falling leaf essences are a vital new type of essence particularly applicable to the needs of the twenty-first century. The understanding of their role in releasing the old and letting go of the past is deeply rooted in the seasonal cycles of the natural world. Ultimately, our ability individually and collectively, to release the accumulated mental, emotional, and physical toxicities from the past, determines to a large extent whether we are able to build a sustainable and better future for ourselves, our families, and society, indeed for the earth as a whole. Falling leaf essences extend, at this pivotal point in history, the opportunity to take a new and better course for the future by releasing the unwanted baggage from the past.

Notes

Chapter 1

1. Rupert Sheldrake, *A New Science of Life: The Hypothesis of Morphic Resonance* (Rochester, Vt.: Park Street Press, 1995).

2. Colin Lessell, *The Biochemic Handbook: A Guide to Using Dr. Schuessler's Biochemic Tissue Salts* (Wellingborough, Northamptonshire: Thorsons, 1984).

3. Clare Harvey and Amanda Cochrane, *The Encyclopaedia of Flower Remedies* (London: Thorsons, 1995).

4. Steve Johnson, *The Essence of Healing: A Guide to the Alaskan Flower, Gem, and Environmental Essences* (Homer, Alaska: Alaskan Flower Essence Project, 1996).

5. Nancy Efraemson and Leonie Hosey, *Shell Essences* (Sutherland, Australia: Shell Essences, 1996).

6. Gurudas, *Gem Elixirs and Vibrational Healing*, vol. 1, channeled by Kevin Ryerson, and vol. 2, channeled by Kevin Ryerson and John Fox (Boulder, Colo.: Cassandra Press, 1985).

7. Irene Dalichow and Mike Booth, *Aura-Soma Healing Through Colour, Plant, and Crystal Energy* (Carlsbad, Calif.: Hay House, 1996).

8. Francis X. King, *Rudolf Steiner and Holistic Medicine: An introduction to the revolutionary ideas of the founder of anthroposophy* (York Beach, Maine: Nicolas Hays, 1987).

Chapter 3

1. Alvin Toffler, *Future Shock* (London: Pan, 1976).

2. Phyllis Krystal, *Cutting the Ties That Bind* (Dorset: Element Books, 1990).

Chapter 8

1. Eric Berne, *Games People Play: The Psychology of Human Relationships* (London: Penguin Books, 1964).

Bibliography

Flower Essences

Bach, Edward. *The Twelve Healers and Other Remedies*. Hereford, England: Flower Remedy Programme, 1989.

Barnao, Vasudeva, and Kadambii Barnao. *Australian Flower Essences for the 21st Century*. Perth: Australian Flower Essence Academy, 1997.

———. *Walkabout Healing Handbook: Healing with the Living Essences of Australian Flowers*. Perth: Australasian Flower Essence Academy, 1990.

Barnard, Julian. *A Guide to the Bach Flower Remedies*. Somerset, England: C. W. Daniel Co. Ltd, 1992.

———. *Patterns of Life Force: A Review of the Life and Work of Dr. Edward Bach and His Discovery of the Flower Remedies*. Worcester, England: Flower Remedy Programme, 1989.

Devi, Lila. *The Essential Flower Essence Handbook*. Nevada City, Calif.: Master's Flower Essences, 1996.

Halpin, Vince. *The Healing Essence of Australian Flowers*. Paddington, Queensland: Unicorn, 1988.

Harvey, Clare, and Amanda Cochrane. *The Encyclopaedia of Flower Remedies*. London: Thorsons, 1995.

Johnson, Steve. *The Essence of Healing: A Guide to the Alsakan Flower, Gem, and Environmental Essences*. Homer, Alaska: Alaskan Flower Essence Project, 1996.

Kemp, C. *Desert Alchemy: Desert Flower Essences Catalog 1992–93*. Tucson, Ariz.: Desert Alchemy, 1992.

Mechthild, Schiffer. *Mastering Bach Flower Therapies*. Rochester, Vt.: Healing Arts Press, 1996.

Shapiro, Jeffrey G. *The Flower Remedy Book*. Calif.: North Atlantic Books, 1999.

Vlamis, Gregory. *Flowers to the Rescue: The Healing Vision of Dr. Edward Bach*. Rochester, Vt.: Healing Arts Press, 1988.

Weeks, Nora. *The Medical Discoveries of Edward Bach, Physician.* New Canaan, Conn.: Keats, 1979.
White, Ian. *Bush Flower Essences.* Singapore: Bantam, 1991.
———. *Bush Flower Healing.* Sydney: Bantam, 1999.

Aura-Soma
Dalichow, Irene, and Mike Booth. *Aura-Soma Healing Through Colour, Plant, and Crystal Energy.* Carlsbad, Calif.: Hay House, 1996.
Wall, Vicky. *The Miracle of Colour Healing: Aura-Soma Therapy as the Mirror of the Soul.* London: Aquarian, 1993.

Cell Salts
Lessell, Colin. *The Biochemic Handbook: A Guide to Using Dr. Schuessler's Biochemic Tissue Salts.* Wellingborough, Northamptonshire: Thorsons, 1984.

Cutting the Ties
Krystal, Phyllis. *Cutting the Ties That Bind.* Dorset: Element Books, 1990.

Gem Elixirs
Efraemson, Nancy, and Leonie Hosey. *Shell Essences.* Sutherland, Australia: Shell Essences, 1996.
Gurudas. *Gem Elixirs and Vibrational Healing,* vol. 1, channeled by Kevin Ryerson, and vol. 2, channeled by Kevin Ryerson and John Fox. Boulder, Colo.: Cassandra Press, 1985.

Homeopathy
Bradford, Thomas. *The Life and Letters of Dr. Samuel Hahnemann.* New Delhi: B. Jain Publishers, 1986.
Callinan, Paul. *Australian Family Homeopathy.* Melbourne, Australia: Viking, Penguin Books, 1995.
Campbell, Anthony. *The Two Faces of Homoeopathy.* London: Robert Hale, 1984.
Castro, Miranda. *The Complete Homoeopathy Handbook.* London: Macmillan, 1990.
Blackie, Dr. Margaret. *Classical Homoeopathy.* Beaconsfield, England: Beaconsfield Publications, 1990.
Clarke, John Henry, M.D. *The Prescriber.* New Delhi: B. Jain Publishers, 1998.
Elmiger, Dr. Jean. *Rediscovering Real Medicine. (The New Horizons of Homoeopathy).* Shaftesbury, Dorset: Element, 1998.
Hahnemann, Samuel. *Materia Medica Pura.* New Delhi: B. Jain Publishers, 1995.
———. *Organon of Medicine.* London: Victor Gollancz, 1989.

Kent, James Tyler. *Lectures on Homoeopathic Philosophy*. Worthing, Sussex: Insight, 1985.

———. *Repertory of the Homeopathic Materia Medica and a Word Index*. 6th American edition. New Delhi: B. Jain Publishers, 1999.

Lockie, Dr. Andrew, and Dr. Nicola Geddes. *The Women's Guide to Homeopathy*. London: Hamish Hamilton Ltd., 1992.

Phatak, Dr. S. R. *Materia Medica of Homeopathic Medicines*. 2nd edition. New Delhi: B. Jain Publishers, 1999.

Sahni, Dr. B. *Transmission of Homoeo Drug Energy from a Distance*. Patna, India: Sahni Publications, 1978.

Vithoulkas, George. *Homeopathy: Medicine of the New Man*. New York: Prentice Hall, 1979.

———. *The Science of Homeopathy*. New York: Grove Press, 1981.

Rudolf Steiner and Anthroposophical Medicine

Carlgren, Frans. *Rudolf Steiner*. Dornach, Switzerland: The Goetheanum School of Spiritual Science, 1972.

Husemann, Friedrich, and Otto Wolff. *The Anthroposophical Approach to Medicine*. Vol. 1. New York: The Anthroposophic Press, 1982.

King, Francis X. *Rudolf Steiner and Holistic Medicine: An introduction to the revolutionary ideas of the founder of anthroposophy*. York Beach, Maine: Nicolas Hays, 1987.

Philosophy and Thinking Relevant to Healing

Ash, David, and Peter Hewitt. *Science of the Gods: Reconciling Mystery & Matter*. Bath, England: Gateway, 1990.

Bach, Marcus. *The World of Serendipity*. Marina del Rey, Calif.: De Vorss & Co., 1970.

Bell, Andrew. *Creative Health*. Auckland: Random House, 1989.

Berne, Eric. *Games People Play. The Psychology of Human Relationships*. London: Penguin, 1964.

Chopra, Deepak. *Quantum Healing: Exploring the Frontiers of Mind/Body Medicine*. New York: Bantam, 1989.

Csikszentmihalyi, Mihaly. *Flow: The Psychology of Happiness*. London: Rider, 1992.

De Bono, Edward. *I Am Right, You Are Wrong. From This to the New Renaissance: From Rock Logic to Water Logic*. England: Penguin, 1991.

———. *Letters to Thinkers: Further Thoughts on Lateral Thinking*. Reading, England: Penguin, 1988.

Gaarder, Jostein. *Sophie's World*. London: Phoenix House, 1995.

Illich, Ivan. *Limits to Medicine. Medical Nemesis: The Expropriation of Health*. Singapore: Penguin, 1984.

Kent, James T. *Lectures on Homoeopathic Philosophy*. Northamptonshire, England: Thorsons, 1984.

Krishna, Gopi. *Ancient Secrets of Kundalini*. Delhi: UBS Publishers' Distributors Ltd, 1995.

Peck, Scott M. *The Road Less Travelled and Beyond*. London: Rider, 1997.

Sheldrake, Rupert. *A New Science of Life: The Hypothesis of Morphic Resonance*. Rochester, Vt.: Park Street Press, 1995.

Toffler, Alvin. *Future Shock*. London: Pan, 1976.

Trees

Adler, Michele. *The Smart Gardeners Guide to Common Names of Plants*. Kew, Victoria: Adland Horticultural, 1994.

Bailey, Liberty H., and Ethel Z. Bailey. *Hortus III: A concise dictionary of plants cultivated in the United States and Canada*. New York: Macmillan, 1976.

Buczacki, Stefan. *Best Foliage Shrubs*. Somerset: Reed International, 1994.

Hibbert, Margaret. *The Aussie Plant Finder*. Balamain, New South Wales: Florilegium, 1998.

Macoboy, Stirling. *What Tree Is That?* Sydney: Lansdowne, 1996.

Rodd, Tony. *The Ultimate Book of Trees and Shrubs for Australian Gardens*. Milsons Point, New South Wales: Random House, 1996.

Spencer, Roger D. *Horticultural Flora of Southeastern Australia*. Volume 1: *Ferns, Conifers & Their Allies*. Sydney: University of New South Wales Press Ltd, 1995.

———. *Horticultural Flora of Southeastern Australia*. Volume 2: *Flowering Plants, Dicotyledons, Part 1*. Sydney: University of New South Wales Press Ltd, 1997.

van Gelderen, Dirk M., Piet C. de Jong, and Herman J. Oterdoom. *Maples of the World*. Balmain, New South Wales: Florilegium, 1994.

Index

About the Author

GRANT LAMBERT WAS BORN in Launceston, Tasmania, in 1956. His schooling was at Scotch College, Launceston. Lambert then completed a bachelor's degree in science with first-class honors in biochemistry at the Australian National University in 1978. A Ph.D. in biochemistry from the same institution followed in 1981.

Dr. Lambert then traveled to England, to take on a postdoctoral research position in genetic engineering at Liverpool University. In 1984 he again moved, this time to Corvallis, Oregon, for a three-year postdoctoral position at Oregon State University. Here he was involved in designing genetically engineered microorganisms for agriculture.

As a result of personal illness, Lambert became interested in natural therapies; he enrolled in a course of study in homeopathy from the Queensland Institute for Natural Science (1988) and received his diploma this was followed in 1989 by similar accreditation in clinical nutrition from the International Academy of Nutrition.

Since 1988, Lambert has worked as a therapist, using homeopathy, flower essences, gem elixirs, and nutritional therapies in his practice. He continues to undertake research into natural medicine and spends considerable time pondering the relationship of science to the intuitive and metaphysical. Rather than abandoning the intellect, Lambert seeks fresh pastures for the intellect to explore, while allowing the intuitive to coexist.

It is from a deep understanding and experience of both conventional science and natural therapies that Lambert writes. He is also an inventor of new essences in natural medicine. To research, develop, and distribute these new essences, Lambert directs a company, Advanced Alchemy Pty. Ltd. The current offerings of the company include all the essences in this book. They may be viewed at www.advanced alchemy.com.au or write P.O. Box 78, Kallista, Victoria 3791, Ausrralia (email: advancedalchemy@ozemail.com.au) for more information.

Dr. Lambert lives and works in the mountains east of Melbourne in a majestic rain forest of mountain ash and tree fern. He shares his home with his wife and two dogs. He is a keen social tennis player, gardener, and international chess player, recently representing Australia in the XIII Correspondence Chess Olympiad.

Books of Related Interest

Hydrosols
The Next Aromatherapy
Suzanne Catty

Aromatherapy Workbook
by Marcel Lavabre

Advanced Aromatherapy
The Science of Essential Oil Therapy
by Kurt Schnaubelt, Ph.D.

Advanced Bach Flower Therapy
A Scientific Approach to Diagnosis and Treatment
Götz Blome, M.D.

The Encyclopedia of Bach Flower Therapy
by Mechthild Scheffer

Vibrational Medicine
The #1 Handbook of Subtle-Energy Therapies
by Richard Gerber, M.D.

The Reflexology Manual
An Easy-to-Use Illustrated Guide to the Healing Zones
of the Hands and Feet
by Pauline Wills

Pilates on the Ball
The World's Most Popular Workout Using the Exercise Ball
by Colleen Craig

Inner Traditions • Bear & Company
P.O. Box 388
Rochester, VT 05767
1-800-246-8648
www.InnerTraditions.com
Or contact your local bookseller